HEINEMANN MEDICAL

STUDENT REVIEWS

GERIATRIC MEDICINE

D1741959

Series editor:
Professor Peter Richards, MA, MD, PhD, FRCP
Professor of Medicine and Dean, St Mary's Hospital
Medical School, University of London

Other titles in the series:
Cancer
Clinical Nutrition
Community Medicine: A Study Guide
Medicine and the Law
Primary Care
Psychology and Medicine

Heinemann Medical Student Reviews

Geriatric Medicine

ANN M. BLACKBURN
AE, MA, MD, MRCP
Consultant Physician and Honorary Senior Lecturer
King's College School of Medicine and
Dentistry, London

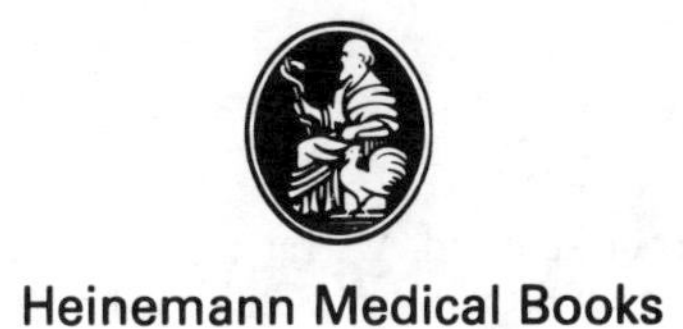

Heinemann Medical Books

Heinemann Medical Books
An imprint of Heinemann Professional Publishing Ltd
Halley Court, Jordan Hill, Oxford OX2 8EJ

OXFORD LONDON SINGAPORE NAIROBI IBADAN KINGSTON

First published 1989

© Ann M. Blackburn 1989

British Library Cataloguing in Publication Data
Blackburn, Ann M.
Geriatric medicine.
1. Geriatrics
I. Title
618.97

ISBN 0 433 00162 3

Photoset by Wilmaset, Birkenhead, Wirral and
printed in Great Britain by Biddles Ltd, Guildford

Contents

Preface vi

Introduction vii

1 Demography and Sociological Aspects of Geriatric Medicine 1
2 Ageing 9
3 Differences in Managing Elderly *vs* Young Patients 16
4 Drug Therapy 28
5 Nutrition 38
6 Confusion and Other Mental Disorders 48
7 Common Forms of Cerebrovascular Disease 63
8 Common Diseases of the Nervous System 75
9 Special Senses—Visual Loss and Deafness 86
10 Falls and Immobility 96
11 Joint Disease and Medical Aspects of Orthopaedic Surgery 108
12 Common Endocrine Problems 121
13 Incontinence and Pressure Sores 136
14 Terminal Care 154

Appendix 1: Areas for Future Research 169
Appendix 2: Training and Career Opportunities 171
Appendix 3: References and Further Reading 173

Index 175

Preface

Although many patients on medical wards are elderly, medical teaching is frequently geared to the specialist interest of the firms concerned. This book is intended to highlight areas of interest for medical students in the care of elderly people. However, no attempt has been made to cover the field of geriatric medicine in a comprehensive manner. Only those areas of concern which are specific to older people are covered; where management of a medical condition is the same as that for a younger adult and well covered in general medical texts, it is omitted here. I hope that this book may also be of interest to people from other medical and paramedical specialities and may enable them to have an appreciation of the many extra components that are required in the care of elderly patients, compared with their younger counterparts.

I acknowledge my thanks to the Office of Population Censuses and Surveys for permission to reproduce Figure 1.1 from *1981 Census: Britain's Elderly Population, Census Guide 1*. Figure 10.1 is taken from a paper by J. H. Sheldon in *Gerontologica Clinica*, 1963 and reproduced by permission of S Karger AG, Basel. Table 5.1 is reproduced by courtesy of Dr C. J. Schorah and the Editor of *Hospital Update*. Table 5.2 is adapted from information published in the *DHSS Report on Health and Social Subjects* No. 15 by permission of the Controller of Her Majesty's Stationery Office. The Norton Scale (Table 13.5) is reproduced from *An investigation of geriatric nursing problems in hospital* by Doreen Norton, Rhoda McLaren and A. N. Exton-Smith, 1962, by permission of The National Corporation for the Care of Old People (Centre for Policy on Ageing), London.

As the majority of elderly people are women, where reference is made to an individual elderly patient in the text, the female gender is used for convenience; similarly, paramedical staff are referred to as female.

I would like to express my thanks to my colleagues at Dulwich Hospital, whose constructive advice and comments on the text have been particularly valuable. Finally, I thank my family and friends, for their forbearance during my writing this work, and to my mother, Mrs Doris Blackburn, for typing the manuscript.

Ann M. Blackburn

Introduction

SCOPE OF GERIATRIC MEDICINE

Elderly people form a substantial proportion of our population today. Population studies demonstrate a disproportionately large rise in the numbers of people over 75 years of age (this group has increased by 12% in the five years since the 1981 Census) and predict a greater increase up to the end of this century. Medical care must therefore adapt to the changing characteristics of the population it aims to serve. Medicine has traditionally been orientated towards the younger patient and to *cure* disease. Disease patterns are changing, as most of the infectious diseases have now been conquered, and the structure of the population is changing—with a reduced infant mortality rate and increased life expectancy. Few diseases at any age can be completely cured; most leave tell-tale 'scars' that can be re-opened later. There are few medical specialities which are unaffected by these changes. The dramatic growth of the elderly population serves as an important challenge to medical students, who will become the doctors of the future.

Geriatric medicine is the branch of general medicine concerned with the many aspects of illness in the elderly population. It has been argued that it is not a speciality in the sense that it does not deal with a single pathology, such as oncology, or a single organ or organ system, such as cardiology. However, the practice of geriatric medicine requires a wide experience of all branches of medicine and the ability to assess and treat patients in the context of their normal home environment. Geriatricians need to be able to distinguish between what are the inevitable effects of ageing and the effects of disease, which therefore require medical treatment. Disease, developing as a result of pathological processes, may either be completely curable or reflect degenerative changes that can be substantially helped by medical means and other rehabilitative endeavours.

The differential diagnosis of the so-called 'geriatric giants', the common presentations of illness in elderly people—confusion, incontinence, falls or instability and immobility—is deceptively wide. Disease may frequently present in an atypical manner in elderly people, who often have multiple pathologies occurring simultaneously. Prescribing for several disease processes occurring together may readily cause unwanted drug interactions. Elderly people, like children, frequently handle drugs in a different manner to younger adults. Knowledge of such factors forms the core of geriatric medicine, but although good clinical skills are essential they are not sufficient alone.

'Whole person medicine' is fundamental to the care of elderly patients. The aim of a geriatrician is to enable every elderly person to live as full and active a life as possible in their own home, or if this is not feasible, in alternative accommodation of their choice. Too often in the past, elderly patients have been seen as passive recipients of care *given* by others. Nothing is more likely to erode their ability and confidence to look after themselves or induce dependence. Medical and nursing care of the elderly sick does not automatically require bed rest and care for every patient, as frequently happens with younger patients. Because unnecessary bed rest is positively dangerous to elderly people, care is typically directed towards enabling them to be as independent as possible, doing as much for themselves as they can, even while they are in hospital. Therefore, unless very sick, they are not nursed in bed all the time, but encouraged to wash and dress themselves whenever possible and move about as they wish in the ward.

Remedial, social and preventative aspects of illness are often as important as purely clinical matters. Rehabilitation, the process of maximizing the patients' potential for recovery after disease (and after trauma or surgery), and the provision of simple aids and appliances in the home environment may transform a difficult existence into a bearable life for an elderly patient. The ability to determine the social and environmental factors of importance in the lives of elderly people is as important as diagnosing their physical and mental conditions. The presence of a flight of stairs to the front door, for example, may be of crucial importance in deciding if an elderly person with mobility problems can return home alone.

The current generation of elderly people have low expectations of their doctors and too often readily accept illness as a 'natural' consequence of their age. Assessment of unreported illness in the elderly community is a large and important area of community medicine, especially of relevance for general practitioners, and may form an extremely satisfying area of preventative care.

The geriatrician cannot be an expert in all these areas of concern in the everyday lives of elderly patients. More than in most other medical

ELIZABETTA

Thanks for your note. Karen + I have gone out. James is in his room. See you Tomorrow

Michael

Thank you for your note! Karen, your father phoned because he was worried about →

Hi!

I'm back, but I went to bed earlier! Sorry, that I have forgotten to phone you! I hope you didn't worry too much!

Goodnight, Elisabeth

specialities, team work is essential, so that expertise from all the paramedical disciplines (physiotherapy, occupational therapy, orthotics, dietetics psychology, speech therapy and social work, to name but a few) can be brought together by the geriatrician and directed towards the welfare of each patient.

Chapter

1

Demography and Sociological Aspects of Geriatric Medicine

CHANGES IN AGE STRUCTURE OF SOCIETY • THE PRESENT ELDERLY POPULATION • ATTITUDES TOWARDS OLD AGE

CHANGES IN AGE STRUCTURE OF SOCIETY

At the beginning of this century in the UK the proportion of the total population older than 65 years was less than 5%, as is still the case now in many underdeveloped countries. Elderly people (when defined as the population of pensionable age, i.e. women aged 60 or over and men aged 65 or over) are a sizeable and growing proportion of our total population. In 1911, less than 3 million people (5.7% of the total population) belonged to this age group, whereas there were nearly 10 million (17.7% of the population) in 1981. Such changes have been brought about by the falling birth rate and reduced mortality in infancy and childhood arising from improvements in public health (housing, sanitation and nutrition), in addition to the reduction in mortality from infectious diseases and the introduction of antibiotics. These changes carry important socio-political implications for public spending on pensions, and for the provision of health and social services.

The proportion of the very old to the total population has also steadily increased. In 1981, out of every twenty elderly people, only one was 85 years or older (1.1% of the population), while five were aged 75–84 years and fourteen were less than 75 years old. In the five years since the 1981 Census, in England and Wales, there has been a rise of 12% in those aged 75 years and older, while the number of people aged 85 and older has increased by 18%. It is calculated over the next 20 years that the numbers of the very elderly will continue to rise steeply (*see* Fig. 1.1). It is this section of the population which makes disproportionately high demands on hospital and general practitioner time and on social services' provisions.

Balance of men and women

Although more male infants are born than female, elderly women outnumber elderly men. For people aged 75 years, there are almost two women for every man, whilst for those aged 85 years, there are approximately three women to every man. Many factors are responsible for this female preponderance in the elderly population and these are related to circumstances that have existed over the past 70 years. Infant mortality was and remains slightly higher for males than females. Many young men were killed at war, or through accidents at work or on the roads. During this century, however, an increasing proportion of women are working outside the home and will therefore be subject to the same work-related hazards, so this trend will become less in the future. Women, until the menopause, enjoy a substantial protection against atherosclerosis and its effects, because of their circulating levels of oestrogens. Many premature deaths are related to the effects of smoking and alcohol, until now associated more with men than women.

Family support

Over the last 20 years, the number of elderly people living alone has doubled. The most recent population Census demonstrated that 30% of elderly people lived alone, 43% lived in private households with another elderly person, while the majority of the remainder lived in households with a younger person, usually a son or daughter.

The average family size has decreased progressively during this century, so that there will be fewer children in the future to look after and help their elderly parents. Children, usually daughters, often carry an extremely heavy burden of care for their elderly parents. This may only become recognized at a time of crisis, or when illness of one party or some other incident occurs, causing a breakdown of the caring relationship. Such situations in the community need to be actively identified, so that strain can be relieved before such a crisis.

Traditionally, the care of parents has been the domain of daughters

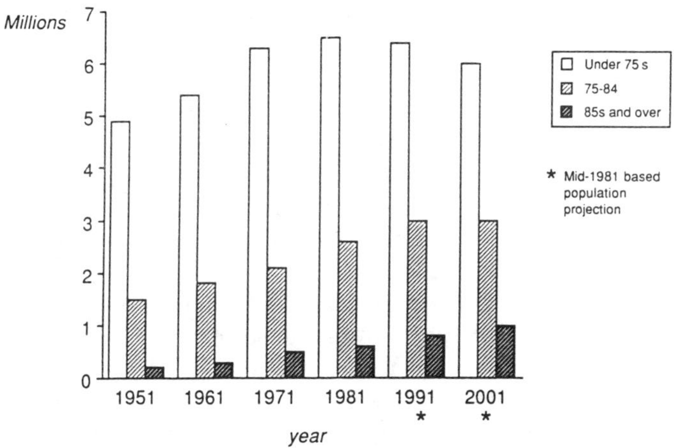

Figure 1.1 Number of the elderly by broad age groups, Great Britain, 1951–2001. Proportion increases have been, and will continue to be, greatest at the oldest ages. *Source: 1981 Census* (ISBN 0 904952 150)

or daughters-in-law who have stayed at home. The proportion of women who go out to work is changing steadily. In 1921, only 8.7% of all women went out of the house to work; by 1976, this applied to 44.3% of the female population. Although the proportion of women who remain unmarried is falling, the divorce rate is increasing. These factors will have a profound effect on the composition of family support for the future elderly population, an effect which is impossible to predict with any accuracy.

Retirement

Society imposes many rules on its individuals, dependent on age. For example, a child must attend school between the ages of 5 and 16 years and cannot buy an alcoholic drink until 18 years old. The age of retirement from employment varies with different jobs; the state pension age in the UK has varied much this century, largely as a result of political and economic considerations. With the increasing longevity of the general population, retirement is a relatively new phenomenon. Since 1940, the state retirement age, at which a government pension may be drawn, has been 60 years for women and 65 years for men. These times are completely arbitrary, not being determined by any biological factors, and they ignore peoples' wide range of abilities at such ages and the wide variations in the demands of their employed work.

Retirement leads to many changes in social and psychological circumstances, which may have deleterious effects on mental health and physical well-being. It is often regarded as a declaration of the unfitness of older people to perform what is required of contemporary citizens and frequently carries the expectation that a retired person will cease all formal and occupational activity. Retirement is associated with loss—loss of finance, as income is often drastically reduced, and loss of status, as a person's position in society, especially for men, is often judged according to their occupation. The reduced income not only reflects the lower status but indeed perpetuates it in today's consumer-orientated society. However tedious employment may be, it orders the day in a structured and purposeful way, which is therefore also lost, as well as providing companionship outside the family circle. Despite these 'losses', the majority of retired people find retirement, especially the early part of it, more enjoyable than work.

Many people at or near their retirement age move to popular retirement areas, thus making their geographical distribution across the country somewhat uneven. In the USA, people tend to migrate from the north to the south of the country, while in the UK, there is a similar movement towards the South Coast and other holiday resorts. For fit elderly people, the move is usually successful, but for those who become disabled, major problems of care arise as there are few resorts which have sufficient resources to provide adequate health and social services for this large proportion of their population.

Isolation

Isolation and loneliness do not invariably occur together. The isolation of many elderly people is a subtle problem which is not readily appreciated and may easily be underestimated by those who are younger. Inevitably, the last few decades of life are associated with bereavement of the spouse and death of other friends and contemporaries. Increasing infirmity, impaired mobility and sensory deprivation (e.g. visual impairment and deafness) may all contribute to substantial isolation, and sometimes, to loneliness and depression. Isolation may also contribute to the development of serious nutritional problems and to mental disorder, especially if compounded by sensory deprivation.

However, isolation depends to a greater extent on an individual's personality and past life-style, and to a lesser extent, on mental and physical health. It has been estimated that 25% of all people aged 70 years and older could be considered isolated and that 14% of those who are housebound or bedfast neither receive visits nor make visits to relatives or friends. Conversely, loneliness may lead to dependence of those who are isolated on other people who happen to come in contact with them. Often, the development of disabling illness, which gives rise to dependence, will ensure that many old people have visits from companions and professionals, who thereby maintain their social lives.

Voluntary organizations in the local community are well placed to ameliorate this problem. They may provide friendly visitors as well as a network of clubs and day centres, usually with the provision of transport to get there. General practitioners, hospital geriatricians and all those working with elderly people should be familiar with the local facilities available to them and even provide stimulation to fill any obvious gaps.

THE PRESENT ELDERLY POPULATION

Living conditions

The majority of older people (95%) live at home in private households, with only one in twenty living in communal establishments, such as homes for the elderly, hostels or hotels. These proportions vary with age, such that many more of the very elderly (19% of those aged 85 years or older) live in communal establishments.

Having lived through times of decreased affluence, and being, as a group, of poor financial means, elderly households are more often without an inside toilet, bathroom, hot water supply or central heating than are younger households. Such environmental factors increase the risk of hypothermia and its consequences.

Elderly married couples rarely require admission to residential care. The strengths of one partner usually compensate for the weaknesses of the other, with both gaining much psychological support from each other. However, when one partner dies, this is particularly traumatic for the survivor, who may have diminished powers of adaptation due to disability or impaired mobility. For these and other reasons, bereavement is associated with increased morbidity and mortality of the remaining partner.

There are many statutory sources of additional finance to improve conditions of living at home, for which elderly people may be eligible. A wide variety of possible Social Security benefits may be explored with the help of the social work department, while for younger elderly people, improvement grants may be appropriate so that their living conditions may be improved.

Community support

Community support is vital for maintaining a reasonable quality of life for the majority of elderly people who live in their own homes. The availability of a home-help service and 'meals on wheels' varies in different parts of the country, but is generally of crucial importance to many elderly people. Indeed, it is not uncommon for elderly people to be admitted to hospital 'unable to cope at home' and, on closer questioning, for it to be found that their home help has gone on holiday or is ill, with no relief having been supplied. Assistance with personal care is often given by district nurses; specific help with bathing may be offered by bath attendants. Incontinence in the home environment can be extremely difficult to manage. If, after full investigation of all possible remediable causes, continence cannot be regained, an incontinence laundry service exists in many areas to wash soiled bed linen. The district nurse may also be able to supply disposable pads and supervise catheter care, where appropriate.

Day centres for elderly people to meet and have a meal together are organized by local authorities and many voluntary organizations. They provide many of the facilities of a social club but often have an important rehabilitative function too, with regular visits from community physiotherapists, occupational therapists and chiropodists. Many elderly people can make their own way to these centres, but others are dependent upon transport facilities, which may be available but are often limited.

There are many voluntary organizations, some local branches of national organizations and some purely arising in a specific locality, which in various ways support elderly people and their carers at home. Some provide a local 'handyman' service, errand service or volunteers to befriend the lonely. For those relatives with a heavy burden of continuously caring for a very disabled elderly man or woman, a 'sitting service' may be a lifeline so that they may have a regular afternoon or evening off to themselves, relieved in the knowledge that their relative is being looked after in their absence. People caring for relatives who have had disabling strokes or who have dementia are often considerably helped by attending carers' support groups.

Services for elderly people must be organized in the knowledge that they will not seek help or demand their rights as readily or vociferously as younger people. However, this does not imply that their wishes are not to be considered or even should be overruled. Everyone in society has the right to live as they wish, but also has the right to refuse help. Only in exceptional, and happily rare, circumstances, are these rights overruled and, in such circumstances, Acts of Parliament have to be invoked (*see* p. 60).

The elderly as a heterogeneous group of people

It is often easy to think of elderly people as a homogeneous group of the population. They certainly have many features in common, which are quite distinct from those of younger people. However, such categorization often denies the recognition of their individual differences and increases the risk of them being classed as a low status, minority group in society. Elderly people show a wide diversity of intellect and physical capabilities and hence of needs. In chronological age alone, they span over four decades of life. More than any other group of people, their individual differences must always be recognized, so that each may be allowed to live as full a life as possible.

ATTITUDES TOWARDS OLD AGE

Ageing is a biological process over which we have virtually no influence, the rate and manner of ageing being determined by an individual's genetic composition. However, 'growing old' can be considered a social process over which we have considerable control. All modern urbanized societies condescend to the values of maturity, but continue to heap honours on the joys of youth. Society, in being materialistic and consumer-orientated, often finds little use for those who no longer contribute to its workforce.

In the UK, 'old age' is conventionally and arbitrarily considered to start at the statutory pension ages: 65 years for men and 60 years for women. To many people, 'growing old' or 'old age' is considered closely related to disability, physical or mental, such that the latter is seen as the inevitable result of the former. Such destructive stereotyping of elderly people, or 'ageism', is as negatively discriminating as racism or sexism. Some loss of abilities is inevitable, but the onset of disability may transform any active, independent person (regardless of age), to one who is inactive and dependent.

The elderly population frequently do themselves a disservice by sharing these ageist attitudes. Many assume that all physical and mental changes are due to 'old age', such that they do not readily or promptly seek help when it is needed. Having lived through the major social upheavals of this century—two World Wars and the Depression of the 1930s—as well as living through a time which has seen a dramatic improvement in basic living standards, their experiences and outlook are often completely different from those of us born more recently. They have experienced lower standards of living and generally have lower expectations, so that they have a more circumscribed view of their 'rights' and hesitate to make demands on society. Whereas we might say 'things could be better', from experience, elderly people often stoically say 'things could be worse'.

It is regrettable that some professionals who are concerned with the care of elderly people may also share these ageist beliefs and fail to distinguish between ageing and disease. 'Well, what do you expect at your age?' is unfortunately still heard in many circles. They may often underestimate the abilities of elderly people and this gives rise to their over-protection, in the mistaken belief that caring means doing *everything* for them. Geriatricians should be an important group to promote opportunities for the well-being and psychological growth of the elderly population, rather than perpetuate society's view of their helplessness and deterioration. Elderly people are not the most privileged in our society; they may have much that is positive to contribute and should therefore be recognized as valued members of society. Perhaps we may consider what Cicero wrote (in his *De Senectute*) in 50 BC, at the age of 63:

> 'If there were no old men there would be no civilised states. Old age is far from being deprived of good council; on the contrary, it has these qualities in the highest degree. States have always been ruined by young men socially and restored by old.'

Chapter

2

Ageing

EFFECTS OF AGEING ON ORGAN SYSTEMS • THEORIES OF AGEING • HUMAN AGEING AND LONGEVITY • PRECOCIOUS AGEING

Death from old age is almost certainly confined to man and those animals he chooses to protect, i.e. domestic and zoo animals. Biological ageing is not generally thought to occur in wild animals. Reproduction is essential for the survival of every species. Most of the recognizable features of ageing occur after the period of reproductive activity has ceased. However, after reaching sexual maturity and cessation of growth, animals accumulate various physiological 'decrements' that increase the likelihood of them dying. Concepts of ageing include many different aspects—social, physiological, morphological, cellular and molecular changes. Ageing may be considered to be that part of a life span during which there is a diminished response to endogenous or exogenous stresses, i.e. when there is a reduction in an animal's ability to cope with stresses imposed upon it by its internal or external environment. Age itself is not a medical diagnosis, but ageing, associated with an increased vulnerability to disease, is inevitable.

EFFECTS OF AGEING ON ORGAN SYSTEMS

It is not always easy to distinguish the changes due to age alone from those due to associated degenerative disease. It has been suggested that any changes which can be considered to be caused by ageing alone must fulfil four criteria: universality, intrinsicality, progressiveness and be deleterious to the individual concerned. In other words, an ageing process must occur in everyone, must not be due to external factors, must be progressive and cause the person some harm. A brief outline of some of the changes considered due to ageing is shown in Table 2.1.

Table 2.1 *Some physiological parameters of body function which alter with age*

Organ system	*Age-related change*
Heart	Diminished cardiac output
	Diminished maximum heart rate
Lungs	Reduced pulmonary elastic recoil (compliance)
	Diminished vital capacity
	Increased residual volume
Gastrointestinal	Reduced secretion of gastric acid
	Reduction in bowel motility
Renal	Reduction in glomerular filtration rate
	Reduction in tubular secretion/reabsorption
Skeletal	Gradual loss of bone substance
	Changes in collagen polymorphism
Endocrine	Reduced carbohydrate tolerance
	Gonadal hormone changes in female at menopause
Central nervous system	Impaired homeostatic functions—tendency to develop hypothermia and postural hypotension
Special senses:	
eye	Alteration in lens composition
	Impaired accommodation (presbyopia)
ear	Degeneration of hair cells in organ of Corti (presbyacusis)
taste	Loss of taste buds
smell	Sense of smell diminished

THEORIES OF AGEING

The ageing process in experimental animals has been studied extensively and there are various theories have been proposed to explain the different aspects of ageing observed. These theories fall into two broad categories: those which state that ageing is in essence genetically programmed, and those that argue that ageing is due to the effects of living. The latter theories propose the accumulation of waste products, or progressive changes in DNA and other macromolecules at the cellular level.

Many theories concentrate on analysis of the disordered cellular morphology known to occur with ageing. Study of immunological changes, which may be genetically determined, could serve to explain the increased susceptibility to infection and the increased incidence of autoimmune disease that are well-recognized in ageing. All theories attempt to explain the gradual decline in certain functions at a cellular level, which result, after a fixed time, in death of the whole organism. Although such theories address the phenomenon of ageing at different levels, the numerous hypotheses may not be mutually exclusive.

Genetically based theories

Life-table statistics show that life span is species-specific, each species having a more or less constant survival curve. This has resulted in attention being focused on genetic mechanisms that might be responsible. Changes in genetic control have therefore been postulated as the common denominator of the ageing process. Some mature cells are totally unable to replicate, e.g. neurones, while others replicate throughout life. Many structural and functional changes occur in normal human cells as they age. Cessation of mitotic activity is only one functional decrement whose genetic control may be similar to that of other age-related events which occur in non-dividing cells.

Cellular mortality and immortality

During the early part of this century, it was found that fibroblasts derived from chick heart tissue could be cultured in vitro serially for an indefinite period. Cell populations were then cultured from a variety of animal species, including man, with similar results. This suggested that there were external constraints on cells in vivo, which prevented them being 'immortal'. However, it was subsequently found that these cultures no longer contained normal cells. Their chromosomal constitution varied from cell to cell and they acquired biochemical properties uncharacteristic of the original cells.

When normal human embryonic fibroblasts were cultured, they were observed to undergo a finite number of serial mitoses or population doublings before they died. Even in the most favourable conditions, death was inevitable after about 50 such doublings. Thus cell death appeared to be an inherent property of the cells themselves and not due to external factors. The doubling potential was inversely related to the age of the donor tissue, such that fibroblasts from a normal adult, for example, only exhibited 14 to 29 doublings. This principle has been confirmed with other human tissues, the number of divisions being related to the cell type. It has been further strengthened by similar work in vivo with experimental animals.

These findings demonstrate that the acquisition of the potential for unlimited cell division or the apparent escape from senescent changes by mammalian cells in vivo or in vitro can only be achieved by somatic cells which have acquired some or all the properties of neoplastic cells.

Immunological theories

The thymic cortex begins to atrophy from puberty onwards and the number of T-lymphocytes starts to fall shortly afterwards. By the seventh decade of life, only 70% of the early adult levels of these cells are seen. The well-recognized reduction in the T-cell-mediated immune response which occurs with age parallels the increasing incidence of autoimmune disease and malignancy. Many of the features of ageing may thus be understood by known changes in the immune system.

Rate of living theory

There appears to be a direct relationship between the life span of different species of animals and their metabolic rates. Both man and mouse expend about 2.9 kJ/g of tissue throughout their lives, but the rate at which this is expended by the mouse is roughly 30 times greater than that of man. The mouse lives 2 to 3 years, compared with man's 60 to 90 year life span. Primates and other mammals have an increasing tendency to longevity, and this is associated with a corresponding increase in those processes which both protect DNA from faulty synthesis and initiate DNA repair.

Theories concerned with the formation of imperfect cells

The *wear and tear theory* suggests that ageing is analogous to the wear and tear effects seen in any working machinery over a period of time. At a cellular level, there is a lack of regeneration to repair the effects of the external environment. The *somatic mutation theory* is supported by the study of chromosomal abnormalities in many tissues, which increase in incidence with increasing age. These chromosomal abnormalities may prevent the normal sequence DNA → RNA → protein synthesis from taking place. Thus cellular division may be impaired or synthesis of abnormal proteins produced which impair cell function.

It is well known that various macromolecules, e.g. proteins and nucleic acids, become less active throughout life because of the introduction of cross linkages between them. Thus the *cross linkage theory* suggests that this is responsible for the observed decline in cell function with age. Similarly, it is recognized that *nucleic acid immobilization* also occurs, i.e. nucleic acid becomes more and more firmly linked to itself or to protein and, it is suggested, is thus less likely to function normally. The *waste products theory* similarly suggests that the accumulation of waste products within the cell, due to, for example, cross linkage changes preventing degradation, act as 'clinker' and interfere with normal cellular function. Inert, lipid–protein complexes have long been observed in cells throughout the body and have been given the name 'age pigment' or lipofuscin. The amount of such complexes increases with age and is thought to originate from the interaction caused by unstable free radicals arising from lipid oxidation products and other lipids or proteins within each cell. There is, however, little evidence to associate the presence of these age pigments with cellular malfunction, especially in the brain, where an accumulation might be expected to show marked correlation with decreased mental capacity.

HUMAN AGEING AND LONGEVITY

Older people, as argued above, are not a homogeneous group. A major hallmark of ageing is the increased heterogeneity between individuals. The rate of ageing appears to vary widely between one individual and another and even in the same individual from one time to another. Functional and chronological age may be differentiated from each another in children by their development milestones. In the same way, not all elderly people are functionally, physiologically, psychologically and socially similar at the same chronological age. For those over 75 years old, their appearance often correlates very poorly with chronological age.

Life expectation in the Western world has increased dramatically over the last two centuries (Table 2.2), but the maximum human life span is virtually unchanged. The reduction of mortality in childhood and the eradication of the infectious diseases, which were previously a scourge to children and young adults, have enabled more people to reach the limit of their fixed life span. Some parts of the world claim great longevity for their inhabitants, but the accuracy of such claims is in doubt. These areas are all at high altitude where the elderly, like the rest of the population, engage in hard physical work and live on a low-protein and -fat diet. However, the greatest age which has been fully documented is 113 years.

Table 2.2 *Expectation of life (in years) at birth and at 60 years of age (in England and Wales) among males (M) and females (F)*

Time period	*At birth*		*At 60 years*	
	M	*F*	*M*	*F*
1838–1854	39.9	41.8	13.5	14.3
1891–1900	44.1	47.7	12.9	14.1
1974–1978	70.0	76.2	15.8	20.4

PRECOCIOUS AGEING

There is a group of rare conditions characterized by the appearances of premature ageing. These follow an autosomal recessive mode of inheritance and have been proposed as models of human ageing. Subjects with *progeria*, for example, show the physical signs of ageing at the end of their first decade of life, which would be typical of their normal counterparts in their seventh decade. Puberty is delayed, usually indefinitely, but mental development is normal. There is severe generalized atherosclerosis and survival beyond two decades is exceptional.

Fibroblasts from individuals with these abnormalities have a shorter life span in vitro and undergo fewer doublings than those from normal adults of the same age. The structure of their collagen is that seen in normal elderly subjects. There is widespread deposition of lipofuscin, adding further biochemical evidence of their premature ageing.

Individuals with *Down's syndrome* also show certain features of accelerated ageing. Down's syndrome is a complex of mental retardation and various physical abnormalities caused by the presence of three copies of chromosome 21 (trisomy) in all cells of the body. Autopsy specimens of the brain show these subjects to have neuropathological signs associated with Alzheimer's disease (senile dementia). This is an area of great interest for research into both ageing and dementia.

Chapter

3

Differences in Managing Elderly *vs* Young Patients

THE PRESENTATION OF DISEASE • HISTORY TAKING • PHYSICAL EXAMINATION • TREATMENT • DAY HOSPITALS

There are many differences to be taken into account when obtaining a history and examining elderly people who are sick, compared with their younger counterparts. More than at any other age, illness will affect the ability of elderly people to live their chosen life-styles. Disease, disability and intellectual function are closely related in enabling or preventing the achievement of that way of life.

THE PRESENTATION OF DISEASE

Multiple pathology

It is common practice with younger patients to gather all the signs and symptoms of illness under one label, one disease or disease process. Such a luxury is rarely possible with an elderly patient. Multiple pathologies co-exist; it is exceptional for an elderly patient to have a single diagnosis. Some conditions, for example generalized osteoarthritis, may not be dominant, whereas others, such as the onset of cardiac failure after a myocardial infarct, may be more relevant in bringing a patient into hospital. As well as considering strictly medical diagnoses, it is useful to have a problem-orientated approach to the many factors affecting the life of each patient. When taking a history, it is often helpful to consider problems under the following headings:

1. Effects of ageing itself, e.g. presbyopia, presbyacusis, affecting the senses of vision and hearing (*see* Chapter 9).
2. Effects of cumulative degenerative disease, e.g. osteoarthritis, peripheral vascular disease.
3. Effects of iatrogenic disability, i.e. the effect of drugs. Multiple pathologies will often result in a wide array of medicines being prescribed. Harmful interactions between drugs may occur in elderly people, as well as there being an increased sensitivity to many drugs, due to altered pharmacokinetic properties (*see* Chapter 4).
4. Effects of the social environment. Medical and social problems are often linked; many elderly people have a well-balanced social network enabling them to manage at home. Patients with severe mental or physical disabilities may gain vital support from a caring spouse, neighbour or home help.
5. The 'final insult'—causing admission. This may be an acute medical episode or sudden loss of social support at home such that life there becomes impossible.

Altered presentation

Disease in elderly patients may present quite differently from that in younger patients. Any symptoms and signs which are present are often muted and less dramatic. Severe, crushing central chest pain, which typically heralds a myocardial infarct in a young subject, is often absent, and instead a recent onset of increased breathlessness is a more frequent complaint announcing this catastrophe in elderly patients. Pneumonia may produce virtually no physical signs, except an increased respiratory rate (and even that may not be present). A urinary tract infection may be 'silent' or present simply with vomiting. Perforation of the large bowel due to diverticular disease, carcinoma, acute appendicitis or peptic ulceration may also be present without agonizing pain, board-like rigidity of the abdominal wall or shock. Pyrexia, drawing attention to infection, seldom reaches the levels seen in younger patients and may be slight enough to be missed altogether.

HISTORY TAKING

As with taking a history from any patient, it is necessary to put an elderly patient at ease by a few general opening remarks. From initial replies to these, one should assess the likely reliability of the history. For instance, it may be possible to ask if the patient knows the name of the hospital where she is or to confirm the means of her arrival there. Further probing of mental awareness and memory may then be necessary, but tact is absolutely essential to avoid giving offence.

Taking a history from an elderly patient often requires considerable patience so that definite problems, if not diagnoses, can be discovered. Commonly, the initial complaint is vague—'gone off her legs', 'collapse' or recurrent falls. Questioning is needed to find the cause of these problems, in the same way as a systematic check-list is often used with younger patients. Possible reasons for vague complaints like these are legion, but vague symptoms should not cause equal vagueness in the mind of the doctor!

History taking may be confounded by the patient's deafness, dysphasia or confusion, which all need to be identified at the outset. Someone who is deaf may well present as confused, answering questions inappropriately. However, this picture may be transformed once a hearing aid is found and put into place! A portable speech amplifier, functioning as a large hearing aid, may be available to help communication if a hearing aid is defective or missing. If conversation still cannot be established, it may often be worth writing a few salient questions on paper, assuming the patients' eyesight allows them to read.

If confused (*see* Mental state below), a detailed history from the patient may be bypassed, but information must be sought elsewhere, from a relative or friend. It is often helpful to seek corroboration of a patient's history from someone living with or near them, who sees how that patient really manages from day to day. Often, people who are mentally alert and orientated, but who have considerable physical disability, may try to deny their problems, even to themselves. Thus, additional information from an independent source can often be important for all patients, but may be vital in the presence of mental confusion or an incomplete or unreliable history from the patient.

The social support of a patient at home is important information to gain. If a patient lives with a spouse, how is he or she? Are 'meals on wheels' brought each day? Do home helps visit? Does the district nurse call and for what purpose? Perhaps there is a son or daughter or next-door neighbour who calls each day; if so, what do they do? Does the patient live in a close-knit community or isolated, with no one to call?

In the presence of physical disability, some details of the patient's home environment are essential. If the home is a flat, how many stairs are needed to reach it, is there a lift, and how often does it work? Are there steps within the home? How accessible are the toilets, etc? Often the rehabilitation of the patient and her successful discharge home is dependent on these kind of details. They are pursued at length by the physiotherapist or occupational therapist, but the doctor needs an idea of possible areas of concern.

PHYSICAL EXAMINATION

The physical examination of every elderly patient must be as thorough as possible as signs of functional impairment are usual in more than one system. If the patient is extremely ill or frail, it may need to be done in several stages, but no system should ever be omitted, even if there are no complaints relating to it, because 'silent' pathology may be discovered and prove to be of vital importance. For example, vision may have deteriorated so gradually due to glaucoma that it has been accepted as 'normal', with obvious consequences. Part or all the examination may need repeating as the extent of a patient's problems become apparent; for example, breathlessness due to cardiac failure during rehabilitation may only become apparent when walking is restored.

Mental state

If there is doubt about the reliability of a patient's history, a quick, simple psychometric test is often helpful, providing a crude discrimination between normal and confused or demented subjects. A commonly used test is the Royal College of Physicians 'mental status questionnaire' of 10 questions designed to measure a patient's orientation, recent memory and conceptual ability (Table 3.1). For those who have lived most of their lives in this country, a score of eight and above is considered normal, whereas less than five denotes severe mental impairment. (NB: simple problems in communication with the patient will totally invalidate this test.) Such a test ignores problems of agnosia or apraxia, and of visuo-spatial perception.

As with physical problems, it may be necessary, if the mental state is impaired, to repeat this assessment later, as the mental state of an

Table 3.1 *Royal College of Physicians 'mental status questionnaire'*

Question	*Score*
1. Patient's age?	1
2. What is the time of day?	1
3. Ask to remember an address for 10 min (e.g. 42, West Street)	1
4. What is the year?	1
5. What is the name of the hospital?	1
6. Recognition of 2 people? (e.g. a doctor and nurse)	1 or 2
7. When were you born?	1
8. When was the First World War?	1
9. Name the reigning monarch?	1
10. Count backwards from 20 to 1 (i.e. 20, 19, 18, etc)	1 or 2
MAXIMUM TOTAL	12

elderly patient is of vital importance to her potential for rehabilitation, future quality of life and eventual place of discharge.

Essential general features

The appearance and general demeanour give important clues. Patients may be cheerful or sad, well presented or dishevelled with a neglected appearance. While some people look young for their age, others look much older.

A patient's *weight* is a valuable baseline to check against further weight loss or gain. Future weight measurement may be required to monitor the reduction of retained fluid in the treatment of cardiac failure or simply to monitor planned dietary restrictions. The *state of hydration* is assessed in a young patient by noting skin turgor, and sometimes, a dry mouth; these signs are unreliable in an elderly person. Skin collagen is reduced by age so that skin turgor, seen by pinching it between the thumb and index finger, is reduced and the skin fold returns slowly to its former position. The presence of sunken eyes is equally unhelpful, while an elderly patient's mouth may be dry because of mouth breathing. The state of hydration may be more readily assessed by attention to the axillae, which are areas of normal sweating, but which in the presence of dehydration are completely dry.

The incidence of arthropathies rises with increasing age, but the *examination of joints*, though time consuming, is necessary if there is any history of joint pain, falls or immobility. Deformities should be noted, and stability and range of movement recorded. The condition of a patient's feet is of fundamental importance to mobility. Hallus valgus, bunions or long, unattended toe-nails are as important in determining mobility and ease in walking as arthritis of the hips or knees. The suitability of footwear is often overlooked yet they may be as functionally disabling as specific problems of the feet themselves.

Breast cancer is the commonest cancer of women and therefore *examination of the breasts* of female patients should be an integral part of every examination.

Before the physical examination is complete, *urine* should be obtained and tested for the presence of *protein, blood* and *glucose*. This can indicate a possible urinary infection, before a mid-stream specimen can be sent to the laboratory for culture; haematuria may point to blood loss from neoplasia arising from anywhere within the urogenital tract. Heavy glycosuria will demonstrate diabetes mellitus, which may accompany a urinary infection and also be responsible for dehydration.

Neurological examination

Assessment of a patient's mental state is an important part of the neurological examination (*see* above). Before beginning a detailed examination, valuable information is gained by asking the patient to walk and observing the gait, or if this is not possible, assessing the control of posture by asking the patient simply to stand or sit unsupported. Muscle mass is much reduced in many elderly people; it is important to distinguish this from focal wasting, indicating neurological disease. Power and coordination in the arms and legs should always be assessed and any asymmetry of movement (including the face) noted.

Muscle tone is often difficult to assess, especially where there is guarding around osteoarthritic joints. There may be a generalized inconsistent hypertonia, only found when the patient is being examined and not affecting voluntary active movements. This phenomenon, called *Gagenhalten* or paratonic rigidity, is thought to represent a form of apraxia in a patient with diffuse cerebral arteriosclerosis. When present, it may sometimes be necessary to replace formal neurological testing with the kind of functional assessment described above. Deep tendon reflexes are often diminished with increasing age, reflecting slowing of conduction in the peripheral nerves.

Sensation, except for vibration sense in the legs, is usually retained with increasing age. Visual acuity can be tested with reading test cards. It is essential to examine the visual fields: the presence of a homonymous hemianopia after a stroke, for example, will be of considerable importance in future management to the nursing and other rehabilitation staff, while a concentric reduction of the fields may point to the presence of glaucoma. Fundoscopy may reveal age-related macular degeneration or the presence of cataracts.

Cardiovascular examination

The response of blood pressure to changing posture is particularly relevant in the examination of an elderly patient. A drop in systolic blood pressure of 20 mmHg or more on rising from a supine position indicates a significant degree of postural hypotension, which may be responsible for dizziness or falls (*see* p. 100). Cardiac rhythm disorders are frequent, but may be episodic. A 24-hour electrocardiograph tracing, when available, is often extremely useful in investigating falls or 'funny turns'. Cardiac murmurs are frequently heard; added heart sounds are of greater significance. Peripheral pulses in the feet should always be sought but may be masked in the presence of peripheral oedema. Oedema of the ankles and lower legs is not a useful indicator of cardiac failure; care must be taken to distinguish it from dependent oedema resulting from immobility, derived from a patient spending most of the day sitting in a chair at home.

Respiratory examination

A raised respiratory rate is an early (and may sometimes be the only) indication of infection in the lower respiratory tract. The presence of kyphoscoliosis causes difficulty in assessing chest movements. Basal crackles alone are not indicators of pulmonary oedema in isolation. They may signify partial collapse of the lower parts of the lungs, due to age-related loss of supporting tissue.

Alimentary tract examination

The condition of the mouth gives valuable information at a glance. The presence of mouth ulcers, fungal infection, the state of teeth, if present, and of the surrounding gums, as well as any maladjustment of dentures, are important to document. Painful dysphagia may be cured by treating oral thrush; weight loss by attention to ill-fitting dentures! Gingivitis may be a focus for septicaemia or bacterial endocarditis.

Palpation of the abdomen, especially if the patient is thin, may reveal a palpable abdominal aorta or show abdominal scars, long forgotten. The presence of faeces in the descending colon can often be felt. A rectal examination is an essential part of every examination and should never be omitted. (Constipation is a common complaint, but diarrhoea may be spurious as a result of faecal impaction; both may be associated with infection in the urine.) In men, the size of the prostate may be noted, and in both sexes, a rectal examination may reveal an unsuspected rectal carcinoma.

TREATMENT

The successful treatment and discharge home of an elderly patient requires the services of many health care professionals. Medical and nursing care can provide specific medical treatment for disease processes such as pneumonia and cardiac failure. The time needed for an elderly person to recover from an acute illness may be longer than in someone younger, but actual time spent in bed must be kept to a minimum. However, many diseases produce chronic disability and treatment of such conditions requires not only their amelioration by drugs, but rehabilitation directed to achieving the optimum functional capacity of patients in their own home environment. For these reasons, a *multidisciplinary approach* is essential to coordinate the many aspects of the treatment of sick elderly patients. This requires effective team work between doctors, nurses and all the paramedical disciplines. For the majority of elderly patients, the skills of physiotherapists and occupational therapists are essential. Speech therapists and social workers have a crucial role in a small group of patients; dentists, dieticians and chiropodists are important in the treatment of others, but may provide considerable assistance with all patients.

Physiotherapy

The role of the physiotherapist is essential in the assessment and treatment of mobility problems, e.g. patients with osteoarthritis or strokes, as well as having a more well-recognized role in the treatment of chest infections. Personal independence implies the ability to move from one place to another at will. Many disease processes of elderly people combine to limit such mobility, e.g. arthritis, cardiovascular and cerebrovascular disease. Physiotherapy aims to maximize functional ability by attention to muscle power, joint movement and coordination between them.

The physiotherapist also plays an important part in teaching and liaising with both the patients and their carers, if they are at home, or with the nursing staff, if in hospital, about the optimum methods of aiding mobility of the patients or of handling them. When walking is no longer possible, it may be feasible to consider teaching the patient to become mobile in a wheelchair, with consequent attention being directed to arm function and the ability to transfer into and out of the chair. If wheelchair independence cannot be achieved, the spouse or other caring relative will require instruction about how to help with such transfers. Alternatively, some patients with limited mobility might be able to manage at home, but cannot venture outside for any distance. Such people can be prevented from being housebound by the provision of a wheelchair for outside use. In such cases, the patients can be taught to propel themselves or a carer can push them.

The physiotherapist is also involved in providing pain relief—for painful joints or muscle strains, by the use of heat, ice, ultrasound or electrical energy (interferential therapy). For intractable pain, transcutaneous nerve stimulation or even, in some departments, acupuncture may be successfully used to diminish pain sensation.

Occupational therapy

The occupational therapist is another key person in rehabilitation of elderly patients. Her role is to look at all areas of patients' lives at home and identify problems in their ability to live their chosen life-styles. Activities of daily living, including independence in self-care, are addressed but leisure activities are also considered. It is vital to ask what the patients see as their problems. Functional independence may be limited by physical or mental disabilities. Cognitive and perceptual assessments, in addition to recognizing patients' motivation and mood, are essential for an occupational therapist to form a realistic appraisal of their problems, and to determine whether they would be able to, and indeed, want to change their behaviour in order to overcome such problems.

In the area of self-care, the occupational therapist needs to determine whether patients can wash and dress themselves. Can they feed themselves and prepare their own meals? She will consider the patient in the physical environment of her own home and may need to visit it, usually accompanied by the patient herself. She may ask questions such as: can the stairs be managed; are rails needed; can the patient reach the toilet easily or would a commode be helpful? If a wheelchair is used in the home, are there any alterations needed in the home (or of the wheelchair) so that all necessary areas in the home can be negotiated?

At the home visit, when key relatives or neighbours may also be invited to attend, normal social interactions may become apparent—to the advantage or disadvantage of the patient. Frail elderly people who live alone may often be supported at home by relatives or neighbours who pop in throughout the day, giving vital assistance, e.g. helping them get out of bed, making drinks or meals, and generally checking that all is well. The willingness of such people, as seen on a home visit, to give this assistance is crucial to the successful return home of many frail elderly patients.

There is a wide range of aids and appliances that can be provided by the Occupational Therapy department to help in the day-to-day life of an elderly person living at home. These may be as simple as replacing buttons on clothing with Velcro fastenings or providing a raised toilet seat, to the provision of a hoist to help the spouse or district nurse lift and transfer an immobile patient from one place to another.

Social work

The social worker involved with elderly people in hospital plays a vital role in liaison between the patient, carers and the various services available in the community. Valuable, independent information may often be obtained by the social worker from the Home Help Service about a patient's home situation. The provision of 'meals on wheels' can be arranged, which may be crucial in the discharge of a frail person who lives alone. Statutory benefits, such as the Attendance Allowance, may not have been claimed where appropriate, because of ignorance; this can be rectified. In certain circumstances, such as the recent registration of blindness, assistance in applying for specific benefits can be given when patients are discharged home.

Various voluntary bodies, e.g. Age Concern, Alzheimer's Disease Society, Parkinson's Disease Society, the Association of Carers (depending upon their availability in the locality), may be contacted to provide additional support and facilities when patients are discharged home. Where available, Day Centres, run by local authorities or voluntary bodies, may provide important social stimulation on a regular basis after discharge. If a patient is unable to go home and there are no long-stay hospital facilities available, the social worker will work closely with the patient and relatives to find her a suitable residential or nursing home.

DAY HOSPITALS

A Day Hospital is a treatment modality which has been well developed by geriatricians. For selected patients, it provides the facilities of a hospital during weekdays, while they return to their own homes in the evenings and at weekends. It is thus both an advantage to patients and economic of staff. Elderly patients may attend a Day Hospital for:

1. Medical and nursing investigation and treatment.
2. Rehabilitation.
3. Maintenance treatment.
4. Social care.

Day Hospitals are part of the hospital service, often sharing facilities with the geriatric rehabilitation departments. All the investigative hospital facilities are therefore available to patients who attend the Day Hospital on one to five days each week. It is therefore suitable for the investigation of less acutely ill people, who do not require round-the-clock nursing care, and may offer continued rehabilitation after a patient has left hospital, perhaps allowing earlier discharge.

Maintenance care may be needed for a small number of physically and socially frail patients, to prevent their deterioration and recurrent admissions to hospital. The regular attendance of a severely disabled patient may also allow sufficient respite to the carer or carers, so that her care can continue at home. Day Hospital attendance, once or twice each week, may also provide respite for the care of patients who would otherwise be unsuitable (because of severe physical or combined mental and physical disabilities) for any other form of day care.

The correct management of a Day Hospital allows it to be a great asset to any geriatric department. Aims for attendance of each patient should be clearly defined by the multidisciplinary team, patients usually attending for a limited period of time. It is generally managed like other wards of in-patients, with regular ward rounds, when patients can be examined, and where both medical and paramedical matters can be discussed and realistic aims of treatment, tailored to each patient, can be formulated and assessed.

Chapter 4

Drug Therapy

DRUG HANDLING IN ELDERLY PEOPLE • OTHER FACTORS CAUSING PROBLEMS WITH DRUG THERAPY • PRESCRIBING FOR ELDERLY PEOPLE • DRUGS WHICH MAY CAUSE PROBLEMS IN ELDERLY PATIENTS

Elderly people are important consumers of drugs. They receive 40% of the UK annual 395 million prescriptions dispensed (1984 figures), although they comprise only 18% of the total population. As discussed in Chapter 3, they suffer more disease and disability than younger people, hence take more drugs for longer periods of time than the general population. The percentage of elderly people taking drugs ranges from 67–87% and, for those on drug therapy, the average number of drugs being taken ranges from 1.7–8.4 per person. Drugs acting on the cardiovascular and on the central nervous systems (CNS) are the most frequently prescribed.

Elderly people are at particular risk of hazardous drug interactions and side-effects both because of the high level of prescribing for their multiple diseases (polypharmacy), and also because of age-related changes in their drug handling. Adverse drug reactions are more common in older patients, and increase with increasing age. They are responsible for, or contribute to, approximately 15% of hospital admissions of elderly people. In addition, mortality from this form of iatrogenic disease rises with increasing age.

DRUG HANDLING IN ELDERLY PEOPLE

Many studies show that the ageing process has a major effect on the response of patients to drugs. Therefore the pharmacokinetic and pharmacodynamic properties of drugs in elderly people are of particular importance.

Drug pharmacokinetics

The intensity and duration of drug action are determined mainly by the concentration of free drug reaching its site of action. The principal factors affecting the amount of free drug at its site of action are its absorption, distribution and elimination, by metabolism or excretion (Table 4.1). Absorption of orally administered drugs is occasionally slower with increasing age, but this is rarely important. For drugs which are highly protein bound, distribution may be altered in the sick elderly patient who has a reduced plasma albumin concentration, thus increasing the proportion of unbound drug and possibly increasing its activity on acute dosage. The distribution volume and hence plasma concentration of both water-soluble and lipid-soluble drugs are affected by age-related changes in body water and fat.

Table 4.1 *Pharmacokinetics: principal changes in elderly patients*

Distribution	↓ body weight ↓ total body water ↑ body fat ↓ plasma albumin
Metabolism	↓ activity of microsomal liver oxidase enzymes ↓ hepatic blood flow
Renal clearance	↓ number of intact nephrons ↓ glomerular filtration and tubular secretion

↓ = decreased; ↑ = increased.

Drugs are mainly excreted by the kidneys or metabolized in the liver, usually to less active or inactive compounds before excretion. Renal excretion and hepatic metabolism become less efficient with advancing age and this may give rise to drug accumulation on regular dosage. As cardiac output decreases with advancing age, systemic perfusion of the liver and kidneys is therefore reduced, and this may have important influences on drug kinetics. Both hepatic blood flow and hepatic function decrease with increasing age. Drugs which undergo first-pass elimination in the liver, such as propranolol and verapamil, are metabolized more slowly in elderly than in younger people. If they are given in the same dose as to the young, higher peak plasma concentrations are likely.

The liver microsomal enzyme systems are chiefly concerned with the metabolism of drugs, and with advancing age, this activity is reduced, while changes in the induction of hepatic microsomal enzymes will alter expected drug interactions. Thus drugs such as the anticonvulsants, some analgesics and anti-inflammatory drugs will, because of their slower metabolism, have higher plasma and tissue levels, longer half-lives and thus have an increased likelihood of causing toxicity.

Alterations in renal physiology are particularly important in the potential of drugs to produce toxicity in elderly patients. Digoxin, a drug that has a narrow margin between safety and efficacy and which is excreted unchanged by the kidneys, is therefore particularly liable to accumulate and cause toxic effects in elderly people. It should therefore always be given in much smaller dosage than in younger subjects and plasma levels checked until the clinical situation is stable.

Drug pharmacodynamics

The changes in intrinsic responsiveness to drugs with increasing age are poorly documented at present. There is evidence that some drugs acting on the CNS produce an enhanced response for a given plasma concentration. Benzodiazepines frequently produce prolonged 'hangover' effects in elderly subjects compared with the young, despite similar plasma concentrations and half-lives in the two groups. Equally, elderly people are more sensitive to warfarin despite its similar pharmacokinetic properties to those in younger subjects. The cardiac effects of isoprenaline and propranolol are less marked, suggesting that tissue responsiveness to these drugs decreases with age. The reasons for these changes are unclear and require further research to define the mechanisms responsible.

Age-related changes in homeostasis

Orthostatic circulatory changes (*see* p. 80), postural stability (*see* p. 96) and autonomic control of bowel and bladder function are impaired with increasing age and are further factors in causing drug-induced iatrogenic disease. An example often seen is that of dependent oedema due to physical immobility, which is incorrectly treated with diuretics. Such treatment may, due to impaired vasomotor responsiveness, result in incontinence because of impaired bladder control and of falls due to postural hypotension.

OTHER FACTORS CAUSING PROBLEMS WITH DRUG THERAPY

Prescribing problems

It is often difficult to resist a patient's requests for a tablet for each new complaint. However, it is essential for doctors to ask themselves if such medication is really necessary. Short-term therapy may often, by default, become long-term. Frequent review of medication is essential to keep the number of medicines taken to a minimum. It is particularly important for general practitioners to undertake long-term supervision of the medication of their elderly patients. Elderly people may sometimes obtain quite different supplies of tablets from their attendance at hospital clinics and from their general practitioner. Unfortunately, such supplies often carry a considerable risk of harmful interactions, thus emphasizing the need for better communication between hospital doctors and general practitioners.

Patient compliance

Compliance is often a major problem with elderly people, especially those who are confused, have poor vision, impaired dexterity, failing memory or who live alone with nobody close by to prompt them. Even for people without such handicaps, drug regimens may be extremely complicated or they may have received such poor instructions about their tablets that they therefore take too many or too few. Drug bottles may be hoarded, with new prescriptions added to and mixed with old, outdated supplies. Compliance may also be threatened if patients find their usual drug formulation has changed colour or shape without any explanation from the prescriber or pharmacist!

PRESCRIBING FOR ELDERLY PEOPLE

Great care is needed in prescribing any medication for elderly people. The dosage of medication may need adjustment to avoid toxicity because of age-related drug pharmacokinetic and pharmacodynamic properties (*see* above). Specific recommendations for drug dosage for elderly people are now required before any new drug, with a prospective market for older patients, can be granted a licence.

The number of different tablets should be kept to a minimum and reviewed at regular intervals. To aid compliance, drug regimens need to be as simple as possible; for example, one tablet a day is more likely to be taken properly than another of similar activity that needs to be taken three times a day. Simple, clear instructions should be given both by the prescribing doctor and the pharmacist. This information is reinforced by the clear labelling of drug containers. Such containers should be easy to open, even for those with arthritic fingers; child-resistant containers, and bubble and blister packs are best avoided.

It is helpful for elderly patients to have a clearly written drug record card, which is kept up to date both by their general practitioner and any hospital doctors also involved in their care (Fig. 4.1). As outlined above, it is regrettable that general practitioners and doctors working in hospital sometimes prescribe for the same elderly patient quite independently and in total ignorance of each other. Better communication between doctors is needed about prescribed medicines to avoid much of the drug-induced iatrogenic disease seen in elderly people.

DRUGS WHICH MAY CAUSE PROBLEMS IN ELDERLY PATIENTS

Drugs acting on the CNS

Hypnotic and sedative drugs

In elderly subjects, hypnotics and sedatives frequently have a more pronounced and longer effect than in younger subjects. The morning after a single dose, elderly subjects may still be drowsy, muddled and unsteady on their feet. Long-term use of such drugs may be responsible for an increased tendency to fall, decreased mobility and incontinence, and should be avoided whenever possible. However, elderly patients may be extremely vociferous in their requests for tablets to 'help their nerves' or to 'help them sleep at night', being unaware of the normal tendency of older people to need fewer hours of sleep and to wake more often through the night. If a doctor decides that such treatment is necessary, the smallest dose possible should be prescribed for a limited

Hospital Clinics attended ______

Name and telephone of family doctor

______ Tel ______

CAMBERWELL HEALTH AUTHORITY
LONDON SE5

Camberwell
HEALTH AUTHORITY LONDON

PERSONAL RECORD FORM FOR MEDICINES

Surname Unit no.
First name Sex
DOB
Address

PLEASE BRING ALL YOUR MEDICATION TO YOUR NEXT OUTPATIENT APPOINTMENT

INSTRUCTIONS

To the Patient

1. Carry this card at all times
2. Show it to your GP/Hospital Doctor/Dentist whenever you visit them
3. Show it to your Retail Pharmacist, when you buy medicines or take a prescription to him.
4. Present this card at the hospital pharmacy when you visit.

To the Doctor

Please enter any changes/additions to the medication prescribed.

To the Pharmacist

Please enter any changes/additions when necessary.

KCH 157

Date	Drug (approved name and strength)	Dose	Directions for taking your medicine				
			At break-fast	At mid-day meal	At evening meal	At bed-time	Additional instructions

Figure 4.1 An example of a patient drug record card. Courtesy of Camberwell Health Authority

time. However if patients have taken such medication, particularly the benzodiazepines, for a long time, such therapy is likely to have induced some degree of dependence and should therefore be reduced very slowly, before being discontinued altogether.

Tricyclic antidepressants

Tricyclics are useful therapeutically for many depressed patients. Plasma levels may vary up to tenfold in elderly patients taking similar doses. It may therefore be necessary to start with very small doses and increase gradually, watching carefully for adverse reactions as well as the anticipated therapeutic effects. The elimination half-lives of the tricyclic antidepressants average from 20 to 35 hours, but in older patients they may be as long as 80 hours. Thus steady-state plasma levels are not reached for two to three weeks. Tricyclics have anticholinergic properties in addition to their primary effect on the noradrenergic neurotransmitter systems of the brain. These properties are responsible for their side-effects: sedation, postural hypotension and dysrhythmias, giving rise to black-outs or light-headedness, urinary retention, constipation as well as the subjectively unpleasant symptoms of a dry mouth and blurred vision. Elderly patients are more susceptible to these side-effects and tolerate them less well than younger patients.

Drugs with dopamine-receptor blocking action

The long-term use of dopamine-receptor blockers, such as phenothiazines (e.g. prochlorperazine), the butyrophenones (e.g. haloperidol), and metoclopramide for dizziness, night sedation and nausea is inappropriate and should be avoided. Side-effects of acute dystonic reactions, drug-induced Parkinsonism and akathisia usually resolve quickly when the offending drug is withdrawn. However the tardive dyskinesias, including orofacial dyskinesias, may take years to resolve and indeed some may be permanent.

Drugs acting on the cardiovascular system

Digoxin

Digoxin is frequently given to elderly patients but the only well-established indication for its use is in the presence of uncontrolled atrial fibrillation, when it must be prescribed with great care. It has one of the highest rates of adverse reactions in the elderly, causing nausea, vomiting, visual disturbance and various types of cardiac dysrhythmia. The incidence of digoxin toxicity has been estimated to be about 25% and is related to the reduced renal function of elderly subjects. Digoxin is less rapidly cleared from the circulation, and consequently higher and more prolonged blood levels are found than in younger subjects. Several studies carried out some time ago, when digoxin prescribing was extremely common, showed that the majority of patients taking digoxin suffered no harm when it was discontinued. The toxicity of digoxin is inversely related to serum potassium levels. Diuretics, especially the thiazide diuretics, tend to cause potassium loss. As patients usually take digoxin together with diuretics to control the fluid retention of congestive cardiac failure, this combination may be particularly hazardous.

Diuretics

It has been estimated that approximately 30% of the elderly population take diuretic tablets regularly. Because of the age-related impairment of vasomotor reflexes and declining renal function, prolonged diuretic therapy may result in excessive depletion of the intravascular volume. This causes the venous return to the heart to fall and in turn the cardiac output to be decreased, leading to postural hypotension (*see* also p. 100), dizziness and falls. In addition, severe electrolyte disturbances, reflecting dehydration, hyponatraemia and further impairment of renal function, may also occur.

Diuretic-induced potassium loss may be corrected by the addition of a potassium-sparing diuretic or potassium supplements. Combination tablets of a loop or thiazide diuretic with a slow-release potassium preparation or a potassium-sparing diuretic are not ideal in respect of the amount of diuretic contained or their ability to maintain normokalaemia. However, they are frequently used with elderly patients to aid compliance. Their use requires careful monitoring of serum electrolytes at regular intervals.

Diuretics are often wrongly prescribed for 'swollen ankles' that reflect dependent oedema rather than congestive cardiac failure. Because of their unsightliness, elderly women complain more frequently about this than elderly men. Attempts should always be made to treat this condition in non-pharmacological ways before using, as a last resort, a weak diuretic. Simple measures, such as elevating the legs as much as possible while sitting, or providing support stockings, will often help considerably.

A diuretic prescription may also reflect the treatment, from years gone by, of mild hypertension; this could now be unnecessary and might therefore be stopped without detriment, or even with benefit, to the patient!

Antihypertensive therapy

There is evidence that long-term treatment of hypertension reduces the incidence of and mortality from myocardial infarction and strokes, but this is less clear-cut in the very elderly, i.e. the over 80s, than in younger subjects. All medication is associated with the risk of side-effects. Such risks are increased in elderly patients with their diminished powers of homeostasis. Centrally acting antihypertensive drugs, such as methyl dopa, and the α-adrenergic blocking drugs, such as prazosin, should not be used in elderly patients because of their marked side-effects. The newer agents, such as the calcium antagonists and angiotensin-converting enzyme (ACE) inhibitors, may be better tolerated. Treatment of hypertension in the individual elderly patient must be carefully assessed and balanced between the risks of no treatment and those of long-term therapy, both with respect to problems of compliance and possible side-effects. Treatment may, for example, be considered more appropriate for someone who is mentally alert and physically active than one of the same age with long-standing mental confusion and immobility.

Drugs acting on the gastrointestinal tract

Antacids

Antacids with a high sodium content may cause fluid retention and worsening of cardiac failure in the presence of heart disease or impaired renal function. As both disorders are common in the elderly, such antacids are best avoided. *Carbenoxolone* has a longer half-life than in younger subjects and is thus more likely, because of its mineralocorticoid activity, to cause sodium retention and hypokalaemia.

Cimetidine

Is excreted largely unchanged by the kidneys. Smaller doses must be used in elderly subjects to compensate for the age-related decline in renal function. It also retards the oxidative phase of hepatic drug metabolism, hence potentiating the effects of many drugs, such as phenytoin and theophylline, which are commonly used by elderly people. Other H_2-antagonists without the potential for these harmful drug interactions are therefore usually prescribed by geriatricians.

Drugs used for joint diseases

Non-steroidal anti-inflammatory drugs (NSAIDs)

These combine analgesic properties with an anti-inflammatory effect and are therefore widely used in the treatment of acute and chronic inflammatory joint diseases. However, NSAIDs may damage the gastric mucosa and impair renal function in some patients. Both effects are related to inhibition of prostaglandin synthesis, but their frequency and severity remain unpredictable. Fluid retention may occur and is sometimes responsible for precipitating cardiac failure, while hypersensitivity reactions are common and bone marrow disorders have been reported.

It is often said that NSAIDs are more likely to cause peptic ulceration, with silent bleeding and perforation, in older than younger patients. There is no doubt that adverse reactions are more likely to be serious, or even fatal, in the older age group. Mild anaemia is often found in patients taking these drugs, but it is unwise to assume the cause is always drug-related. Gastric irritation or ulceration may equally co-exist with a slowly bleeding colonic or rectal carcinoma, which requires treatment in its own right.

Antibiotics

Antibiotics that are excreted unchanged by the kidneys, e.g. the *aminoglycosides*, need to be used in lower doses in elderly patients than their younger counterparts. Renal damage and ototoxicity is prevented by careful monitoring of drug levels in the blood at peak and trough times. Gentamicin should generally be avoided in elderly patients, except in extreme circumstances of bacterial resistance.

Chapter

5

Nutrition

SPECIFIC NUTRIENT DEFICIENCIES • MULTIPLE NUTRIENT DEFICIENCIES • ALCOHOLISM • DEMENTIA • IDENTIFICATION AND CARE OF HIGH-RISK GROUPS

Clinical malnutrition is uncommon in industrialized Western countries. However, subclinical malnutrition, consequent upon the poor diet of many elderly people, may be implicated in the production of non-specific symptoms or a reduced resistance to disease and other stresses. Assessment of the nutrition of any patient is complex: factors such as food intake, nutritional status, physical activity *vs.* energy expenditure all need to be considered. The nutritional status of a patient, encompassing anthropometric, biochemical and clinical assessment, is often difficult to define and measure. Differences in the average values of selected indices of nutrition in healthy and sick elderly women are shown in Table 5.1, and compared with a younger group.

Table 5.1 *Average values for indices of nutrition in different groups of women* (after Schorah and Morgan (1985))

Subject group	*Plasma composition*			*Physical (body) composition*	
	albumin (g/l)	*vitamin C (mg/l)*	*folate (μg/l)*	*fat-free mass (kg)*	*triceps skin-fold thickness (mm)*
Healthy <65 yrs	43	9.5	6.2	44	16.6
Healthy >65 yrs	39	4.9	3.3	41	18.8
Sick >65 yrs with:					
chronic illness	37	3.5	2.9	34	9.5
acute illness	35	2.8	3.2	35	9.9

Although the anthropometric norms of elderly people are calculated to be less than those of younger people, elderly people with values well below normal are likely to be poorly nourished. Biochemical values of nutritional state also vary with age, but some may also vary in the presence of disease. Serum albumin may be abnormally low, either due to reduced protein intake or increased catabolism secondary to disease. Anaemia is common, but there are numerous causes to be considered apart from dietary insufficiency. Disorders of nutrition and disease are closely related; each may be implicated in the production of the other.

SPECIFIC NUTRIENT DEFICIENCIES

The recommended daily amounts of food energy and various nutrients for elderly people over 75 years of age are shown in Table 5.2.

Table 5.2 *Recommended daily amounts of food energy and nutrients for elderly people over 75 years old in the UK* (from DHSS Report on Health and Social Subjects No. 15. HMSO (1979))

	Men	*Women*
Energy (kcal)	2150	1680
Protein (g)	54	42
Iron (mg)	10	10
Calcium (mg)	500	500
Vitamin C (mg)	30	30
Vitamin A (μg retinol equivalents)	750	750
Thiamine (mg) (vitamin B_1)	0.9	0.7
Riboflavine (mg) (vitamin B_2)	1.6	1.3
Nicotinic acid (mg equivalents)	18	15
Vitamin D (μg) (cholecalciferol)	10	10

Vitamin C (ascorbic acid)

Many elderly people, for economic or social reasons, have less than the recommended daily amount of this vitamin (30 mg) in their diet. Accordingly, mean plasma and leucocyte vitamin C concentrations are lower in elderly than in younger people (Table 5.1). However, frank cases of scurvy are not common but may be seen occasionally in elderly men living alone. Some of the earliest signs of clinical scurvy, such as bruising, anaemia, behavioural changes, lethargy and muscle weakness, are common symptoms of many sick, elderly people. The presence of sheet haemorrhages, usually on the legs, follicular haemorrhages and stunted, curled body hairs are more diagnostic signs. The diagnosis is confirmed by measuring leucocyte ascorbic-acid levels, a test unfortunately not universally available.

Folic acid

Folic acid, concentrated in green vegetables and liver, may be deficient because of reduced intake from a poor diet. Its absorption may be impaired as part of a malabsorption state (*see* below).

Folic acid deficiency, as demonstrated by low red-cell folate levels, is common in elderly patients and frequently gives rise to anaemia. When this deficiency occurs alone or in combination with vitamin B_{12} deficiency, a macrocytic blood film is seen, arising from a megaloblastic bone marrow. It is always advisable, in any patient with a macrocytic anaemia, to measure both folic acid and vitamin B_{12} levels. In patients with both folic acid and vitamin B_{12} deficiencies, subacute combined degeneration of the cord may be precipitated by folic acid administration alone. A clear-cut macrocytic anaemia will not be found if there is also a deficiency of iron, and in such cases, levels of all three haematinics will need to be measured. Deficiency of folic acid is readily treated orally by folic acid tablets, although parenteral administration is also available.

Vitamin B_{12} and pernicious anaemia

Vitamin B_{12} deficiency is hardly ever due to simple dietary deficiency. Although it may be seen in vegans, it is usually due to malabsorption (*see* below). Pernicious anaemia, a specific type of malabsorption and the commonest type of megaloblastic anaemia, is essentially a disease of later life. It is estimated to occur in 1% of the general population over the age of 60. The cause is a failure of the gastric parietal cells to produce both gastric acid and the transport protein 'intrinsic factor', probably as a result of an autoimmune gastritis. An association with other autoimmune diseases, especially the autoimmune thyroid disorders and rheumatoid arthritis, is often observed.

The anaemia has an insidious onset and may therefore be quite severe before it is noticed. Common symptoms are glossitis, anorexia and cardiac failure (secondary to the severe anaemia). Occasionally, mental changes, confusion or psychoses may occur. Rarely, the complex of neurological problems of subacute combined degeneration of the cord may present: paraesthesiae and unsteadiness may be accompanied by signs of peripheral neuropathy, while paraplegia and sensory ataxia may indicate pyramidal and posterior column lesions. The anaemia may be associated with anorexia, nausea and weight loss—suggestive of a gastric neoplasm. This tumour may co-exist, as its incidence is much higher in patients with pernicious anaemia than in the general population.

The diagnosis of pernicious anaemia is made by finding a macrocytic anaemia, with the mean corpuscular volume between 110 and 140 cubic microns (normal range 75–95), a low serum B_{12} and megaloblastic erythropoietic changes in the bone marrow. Various additional tests have been devised to demonstrate impaired B_{12} absorption. The Schilling urinary excretion test measures the urinary excretion of vitamin B_{12} after it has been given alone or combined with intrinsic factor. However, a 24-hour urine sample is needed for this test, which is fraught with possible errors in collection with elderly subjects. This disadvantage is removed using the Dicopac test, a double radioisotope urinary excretion test.

Treatment is by intramuscular injections with hydroxycobalamin (Neo-cytamen) and must be continued for life. Initial doses, 1000 μg on alternate days for five days, are needed to replenish body stores of vitamin B_{12}, followed by similar maintenance doses every two months thereafter. Failure to observe a reticulocyte response after five days may occur if folic acid or iron stores are also low and needing replacement at the same time. Similarly, patients with coincidental hypothyroidism will not respond until thyroxine therapy is begun.

Iron

Iron deficiency is very common in the elderly population, whether accompanied by anaemia or not. Inadequate dietary intake may be an important aetiological factor. Elderly women may be particularly vulnerable to dietary deficiency, often having low iron stores due to prior blood loss from menstruation and child-bearing in their earlier years. Elderly men living alone may also be at risk if they neglect their diet.

Chronic gastrointestinal blood loss is a more likely cause of iron deficiency anaemia than dietary deficiency and should always be considered and investigated as appropriate. Drugs such as aspirin and the non-steroidal anti-inflammatory agents (*see* Chapter 4) may also cause chronic bleeding from the stomach. However, the well-known propensity for multiple pathology in elderly people may be responsible for any anaemia having more than one cause.

Iron deficiency is diagnosed by demonstrating a hypochromic, microcytic anaemia and confirmed by finding a low serum iron and raised serum iron-binding capacity. Serum ferritin mirrors the body iron stores, being low only when there is deficiency of iron, and is becoming increasingly measured to detect iron deficiency. Numerous preparations of oral iron supplements are available to restore the haemoglobin and iron stores to normal. However, even if further iron loss is halted, this may take many months. If there is gastric intolerance or compliance problems, or alternatively if a rapid response is needed, parenteral routes for iron therapy, or even a blood transfusion, may occasionally be necessary.

Calcium

The precise role of calcium in the diet of elderly people in relation to their known loss of bone mass remains ill-defined and controversial. Peak bone mass is achieved at the age of 30–35 years, after which the mineral content of the skeleton gradually declines. It may be that the risks of osteoporotic fractures in old age are determined by the peak bone mass achieved 40 years earlier. Calcium balance is affected by age, illness, exercise and other dietary nutrients. Endocrine manipulation and calcium supplementation are known to affect bone density at the time of the menopause but their value in the elderly population is speculative.

Vitamin D

Dietary deficiency of foods containing vitamin D, i.e. dairy products, fortified margarine and fish such as herring, sardine and salmon, may lead to osteomalacia (*see* Chapter 12). Of greater importance is the endogenous production of 25-hydroxy cholecalciferol by exposure of the skin to sunlight, which may be impaired in housebound subjects, causing them to have osteomalacia.

MULTIPLE NUTRIENT DEFICIENCIES

Malabsorption syndromes

As the mucosa of the small bowel is responsible for absorption of nutrients from the diet, any disease process or structural abnormality of the upper gastrointestinal tract is liable to interfere with the absorption of multiple nutrients and produce a malabsorption state. Malabsorption is not uncommon in the elderly population but in the absence of signs of gross disease, symptoms are frequently non-specific and likely to be dismissed as simply 'due to age'. Anaemia is the most frequent presenting symptom, while muscle weakness and bone pain from osteomalacia may also occur. Causes of malabsorption in elderly people are shown in Table 5.3.

Table 5.3 *Causes of malabsorption*

Associated with gastrointestinal disease

1. *Gastric* lesions, e.g. chronic atrophic gastritis, pernicious anaemia, partial/total gastrectomy
2. *Intestinal*, e.g. coeliac disease, Crohn's disease, jejunal resection, conditions causing bacterial overgrowth*, infection (e.g. *Giardia lamblia*), chronic mesenteric ischaemia
3. *Pancreatic* disease (and associated steatorrhoea)
4. *Hepatic* disease

Associated with systemic disease
Drug-induced, e.g. cytotoxic and anti-folate drugs

* i.e. following gastrectomy, idiopathic hypo/achlorhydria, formation of surgical blind loops, duodenal and jejunal diverticula, fistulae

Malabsorption after gastric surgery

With partial gastrectomy for peptic ulceration, a large part of the acid-secreting section of the stomach is removed, as is the tissue that normally secretes intrinsic factor, necessary for vitamin B_{12} absorption. Hypochlorhydria develops with increasing frequency in elderly people and gastric surgery may further reduce acid production. Pernicious anaemia may develop in 5% of such patients after 10 years, but invariably occurs within 3 to 4 years after total gastrectomy, unless replacement vitamin B_{12} is instituted.

Iron deficiency anaemia is also frequent and may develop in up to

50% of patients after various types of gastrectomy. Reduced intake of iron, failure to absorb it because of duodenal by-pass or bleeding from the mucosa adjacent to the anastomosis may all be responsible. Osteomalacia may develop 5 to 20 years after gastrectomy and is believed to be due to a diminished intake and/or defective absorption of vitamin D.

Malabsorption associated with small bowel pathology

Conditions that distort the structure and function of the villi in the jejunum or ileum will also cause malabsorption of multiple nutrients, depending upon the site of damage. Crohn's disease, gluten-sensitive enteropathy or surgical resection of the small bowel may cause vitamin B_{12} or folic acid deficiencies. Crohn's disease may be diagnosed for the first time in elderly patients, in whom it is more often localized to the large bowel than in younger patients.

Bacterial overgrowth in the small bowel is frequently responsible for multi-vitamin deficiencies, especially of vitamin B_{12}. It may occur after surgery or pathological alterations in the bowel anatomy, or secondary to the age-related reduction of acid production by the stomach. These opportunistic bacteria may damage the intestinal mucosa and reduce its absorptive capacity or directly compete for nutrients with the host. Bile salt metabolism may also be upset, with resultant interference in absorption of fat and fat-soluble vitamins. Broad-spectrum antibiotics are extremely effective treatment for this condition.

Chronic intestinal ischaemia may cause global dysfunction of the small bowel. It commonly causes pain after eating but, unlike peptic ulceration, symptoms are not alleviated by the administration of antacids. The radiological presence of vascular calcification within the abdomen, indicating severe atherosclerosis (within the abdomen), gives support to this diagnosis. The diagnosis may be confirmed by arteriography, but as treatment is conservative, this is hardly ever performed.

Malabsorption associated with pancreatic and biliary disease

Pancreatic disease and any hepatic disease causing biliary strictures will be associated with steatorrhoea, and malabsorption of fat and the fat-soluble vitamins, A, D, E and K. Osteomalacia will result from failure of hepatic metabolism of vitamin D, in addition to failure of its absorption. Levels of folic acid and vitamin B_{12}, which normally undergo an enterohepatic circulation, will also be reduced.

Malabsorption associated with systemic diseases and drugs

Malabsorption may also be a manifestation of systemic diseases such as amyloidosis, rheumatoid arthritis and chronic congestive cardiac failure. Some drugs may be incriminated in producing malabsorption, e.g. the cytotoxic agents, colchicine and neomycin. Others may interfere specifically with one nutrient, e.g. the anticonvulsants, trimethoprim and the anti-folate cytotoxic agent, methotrexate, all antagonize folic acid metabolism.

ALCOHOLISM

Alcoholism is becoming increasingly recognized in elderly patients. In studies from the USA, the peak incidence appears to be between 65 and 75 years of age with a male: female ratio of 3:2. As with younger patients, excess consumption of alcohol is seldom admitted to initially by elderly patients. It may be the continuation of life-long alcohol abuse or may be a more recent development, with an increased consumption in later life being an attempt to counteract depression, anxiety or general unhappiness.

Alcoholism is frequently associated with a reduced food intake and, in time, generalized malnutrition. Most vitamins will be taken in less than the daily recommended amounts. Korsakoff's syndrome, an amnestic syndrome with alterations in memory and new learning, is related to thiamine deficiency and may be seen in alcoholic patients.

Iron deficiency anaemia may result from blood loss following gastritis or haemorrhage from oesophageal varices, a consequence of portal hypertension and cirrhosis. Alcoholism may be associated with chronic pancreatitis and steatorrhoea. Impairment in absorption of fat and of the fat-soluble vitamins may cause osteomalacia (*see* above). Macrocytosis is common and usually not associated with deficiencies of folic acid or vitamin B_{12}; it is thought to be a consequence of a direct toxic effect of alcohol on the bone marrow.

DEMENTIA

It is well known that elderly women with dementia have lower body weights than elderly women with affective disorders and schizophrenia. Elderly people with severe dementia are likely to be found on long-stay hospital wards. Such patients rarely show evidence of malnutrition, although low body weight is not related to the length of hospital stay. Patients in psychogeriatric wards tend to have lower energy intakes when compared with matched groups in the community; they may also expend more energy as a result of restlessness.

The relationship between nutrition and the cerebral metabolism of demented subjects is complex. Many vitamins of the B group, especially thiamine, nicotinic acid, pyridoxine, folic acid and B_{12}, play an important role in brain metabolism, and their deficiency is associated with various neurological and psychological diseases. Evidence is conflicting as to whether most of these associations are due to a cause or an effect relationship.

IDENTIFICATION AND CARE OF HIGH-RISK GROUPS

Several large surveys of elderly people living at home have been carried out; these give the proportions of those considered to be clinically malnourished as between 6 and 8%. This percentage is increased in elderly patients with chronic disabling diseases or those who are living in institutions. Chronic disease may affect the absorption, metabolism and distribution of nutrients. Other factors related to under-nutrition in the elderly population are shown in Table 5.4.

Table 5.4 *Factors associated with malnutrition in elderly people*

Medical	
(metabolic causes)	Chronic illness, e.g. chronic bronchitis, emphysema, gastrointestinal disease, partial gastrectomy
(poor intake)	Poor dentition (edentulous or not using dentures while eating)
	Difficulty in swallowing
	Mental impairment: depression, dementia, apathy
	Housebound (poor mobility)
Social	
(poor intake)	Loneliness and social isolation
	Bereavement
	No or few regular cooked meals
	Alcoholism
	Living alone (for men only)

Elderly patients at risk of dietary deficiency are those with diseases that have metabolic consequences affecting the utilization or absorption of nutrients, e.g. gastrointestinal disease, malignancy and infection. However, other elderly subjects may equally be at risk of subnutrition because of poor food intake, a low income, living alone or being institutionalized. If living at home, decreased mobility of elderly subjects may result in their having a poor diet. Chronic mental or physical disease may be associated with a poor appetite, alterations in taste, dental problems or behavioural changes, which will all result in a poor dietary intake.

As only a minority of old people suffer from obvious malnutrition, it is necessary to identify those at risk. In the community, this is the task of the primary care team, supported wherever possible by a health visitor or specialized geriatric visitor. Thereafter, the dietician may have a part to play in providing advice and designing and distributing booklets for later reference. This is most easily organized in day centres, lunch clubs and day hospitals.

If total protein and calorie intakes are low, the diet may be supplemented by arranging delivery of pre-cooked meals from the 'meals on wheels' service, at least four times each week. However, there are potential problems, such as loss of nutrient value during distribution and ensuring that the meals are actually eaten. Meals served at lunch clubs, day centres and day hospitals are more likely to be effective because they are eaten with others. Relatives should also be given advice from a dietician or health visitor on specific nutritional problems.

For patients with biochemical evidence of osteomalacia, there is no doubt that regular calciferol is beneficial. Alcoholics with or without evidence of the thiamine–deficiency states Wernicke's encephalopathy and Korsakoff's psychosis, will benefit from injections of vitamin B complex. Vitamin C supplements may be useful in patients to accelerate healing of surgical wounds and pressure sores, while liquid protein supplements have been shown to counteract the catabolic effects of trauma in patients with hip fractures. However, whether nutritional supplements will benefit the many ketotic and acutely ill elderly patients seen in hospital remains an open question at present.

Chapter

6

Confusion and Other Mental Disorders

TYPES OF CONFUSION • DEMENTIA • OTHER PSYCHIATRIC DISORDERS OF ELDERLY PEOPLE • LEGAL ASPECTS OF MENTAL DISORDER

Confusion is a term understood in general terms by medical and lay people alike and describes the symptoms rather than a diagnosis of disordered cerebral function. It is important to understand because of its great prevalence in the sick elderly population and because it is an important pointer to physical illness, much of which is remediable. It may be described as a varying disorder of awareness associated with:

1. Intellectual impairment, e.g. disorientation, defects in attention and grasp, faulty perception and mis-identification, hallucinations and illusions, impairment of judgement and insight.
2. Emotional upset, e.g. fear, bewilderment, rage, euphoria.
3. Disturbed behaviour, e.g. restlessness, noisiness, aggression and apathy.

It is important to distinguish a recent onset of confusion from long-standing confusion as they have different options for treatment and, usually, a totally different prognosis.

TYPES OF CONFUSION

Confusion of recent onset

The ageing brain is particularly vulnerable to acute impairment of its function by a variety of circumstances, listed in Table 6.1. When confusion is of recent onset, it is particularly likely to represent a confusional state due to underlying physical disease. Often the confusion starts abruptly with fluctuation in the level of consciousness, but such information is only obtained when there is a relative or neighbour available who is able to act as a witness. Confusion serves as a non-specific presentation of physical disease, the symptoms and signs of which may be slight or entirely lacking. This situation equally applies when a mildly demented patient shows a sudden worsening in the degree of her confusion. Indeed, pre-existing dementia increases an elderly person's vulnerability to the development of an acute confusional state.

Table 6.1 *Causes of acute confusion**

Infections	Especially pneumonia, pyelonephritis, neurosyphilis
Cerebral hypoxia	e.g. Following myocardial infarct, cardiac failure, dysrhythmias, respiratory failure, severe anaemia, post-ictal and post-cerebrovascular events
Carcinomatosis	
Metabolic causes	e.g. Hypoglycaemia, diabetic ketoacidosis, uraemia, hyperparathyroidism, hypoparathyroidism, water intoxication, water depletion, hypokalaemia, liver failure, myxoedema, thyrotoxicosis (especially 'apathetic' type)
Drug-induced	Especially alcohol, barbiturates, digoxin, L-dopa, benzhexol
Depression	'Pseudo-dementia'
Environmental and social change	e.g. Bereavement, social upheaval or disaster, or other abrupt change of environment
Head injury	
Nutritional disorders (rarely)	e.g. Pellagra, scurvy, vitamin B_{12} and folic acid deficiency

* A term with multiple synonyms including delirium and toxic confusional state

The most common causes of acute confusion are the acute infections, particularly pneumonia, respiratory and urinary infection, cardiac failure, carcinomatosis (in the absence of cerebral metastases) and drugs (especially those with anti-cholinergic properties). In such diseases, the cause of the confusion is outside the brain, with functional, but no structural cerebral changes being detected. Management should therefore be directed towards determining the cause of confusion and providing specific treatment for that, rather than giving non-specific therapy directed to the confusion alone.

General therapeutic measures include the withdrawal of all inessential medication, the correction of dehydration or electrolyte imbalance, when present, and the minimum use of sedation (if not its total avoidance).

Persistent and long-standing confusion

Long-standing confusion (sometimes called chronic brain failure), particularly if it progressively worsens, is most often due to dementia but can represent a confusional state due to physical disease. Other diseases of the central nervous system, with organic brain pathology, may also rarely cause this clinical picture (*see* below) and therefore need to be considered. Such intrinsic causes of brain failure with structural abnormalities contrast with those mentioned above, which have no demonstrable structural changes.

DEMENTIA

Definition and types

Dementia is a clinical syndrome where there is a diffuse failure of memory, intellect and personality. It has been defined as a global disturbance of higher cortical functions including memory, problem-solving ability, performance of learned perceptual and motor skills, orientation in time and place, correct use of social skills and control of emotional reactions, in the absence of gross clouding of consciousness. It usually has an insidious onset and is slowly progressive. It is rare below the age of 45 years but affects one in twenty people over the age of 65 years and one in four of those over 80 years old. Dementia is more destructive of a person's quality of life than any purely physical disability, although institutional care is only required in the most severe cases. Dementia is of particular importance for doctors to recognize because, with the growing elderly population, the numbers of such patients are rising and their care is making ever increasing demands on the health and welfare services.

Alzheimer's disease

Alzheimer's disease (also known as senile dementia of the Alzheimer's type; SDAT) is the commonest type of dementia in old age and accounts for about 50% of all cases. The diagnosis is suggested by a slowly progressive decline in mental capacity, with memory impairment a common early feature. It is a disease that has excited much neurochemical and genetic research, but as yet no clues for its treatment. The definitive diagnosis is histological, made at post mortem examination, when characteristic neurofibrillary tangles and senile plaques within the neocortex can be observed. The computerized tomography (CT) scan may show a variable degree of cortical atrophy, but this does not correlate well with the cognitive impairment.

Multi-infarct dementia

Multi-infarct dementia, accounting for 20% of all patients with dementia, tends to have a history of more sudden onset and step-wise deterioration in mental impairment, often associated with minor strokes and the presence of focal neurological signs and hypertension. It is thought to be caused by cerebrovascular disease and was previously called 'atherosclerotic dementia', although the terms vascular or multi-infarct dementia are now preferred. Incontinence commonly occurs early in the disease progression. Pathologically, disseminated cortical softening is observed, due to multiple small infarcts, which can be seen on CT scanning. It may be difficult at times to distinguish between the Alzheimer's and multi-infarct dementia and, indeed, both may be found together at post mortem examination (in 20% of cases).

Dementia associated with other neurological diseases

Dementia may be associated with Parkinsonism and other degenerative neurological conditions, such as Huntington's chorea and Pick's disease. It may be a consequence of viral infections, (e.g. Jakob–Creutzfeldt disease and infection with the recently discovered human immunodeficiency virus) as well as long-standing normal pressure hydrocephalus.

Diagnosis of dementia

Both the history and examination of any patient suspected of having dementia need to elicit evidence of a diffuse and progressive failure of memory, intellect and personality.

Conversation with patients suffering from dementia needs, in as natural a way as possible, to determine whether they can give a good account of their circumstances—for example, how they manage at home and how they spend their time. This information, however, should always be corroborated by a relative or close friend, to whom more direct questions can be directed to determine the patient's social competence. Short- and long-term memory may be tested, as may orientation, calculating ability and language competence. Points in the history that are important to obtain from a second person include ascertaining the rate of evolution of the mental disturbance, any evidence of failing intellect or social capacity, the patient's previous personality and any mood changes. Enquiry should also be made about any major social upheavals in the patient's recent past, any history of head injury, as well as the possible co-existence of physical symptoms.

Gradually developing mental changes can be subtle and not always noticed at first by close relatives. Evidence of these changes may include a slight decline in appearance or personal hygiene, a decline in the ability to handle money or minor offences against the social code. It may be difficult in the early stages to distinguish such changes from personal eccentricity.

Formal psychometric tests are useful screening devices which measure orientation, recent memory and conceptual ability. A short one is the mental status questionnaire of the Royal College of Physicians (*see* Table 3.1). However, it is important not to subject patients to a barrage of questions which can cause offence. The remaining part of the physical examination may be almost normal in the early stages of the disease.

As dementia progresses, the gait often slows down and becomes shuffling, the posture bent forward and reflexes of infancy reappear. A pseudo-bulbar palsy may sometimes be present, i.e. a bilateral upper motor neurone lesion affecting the bulbar innervated muscles, caused (in this case) by cerebrovascular disease and which may be responsible for slurring of speech and difficulty in swallowing. A variety of focal brain syndromes may be seen in some (multi-infarct) demented patients, while the three As—agnosia, apraxia and aphasia—are common in those (with Alzheimer's type) who are severely affected.

Differential diagnosis

It is essential that any patient suspected of having dementia should be investigated to exclude other physical and mental illness causing cognitive impairment, which may masquerade as chronic confusion (*see* Table 6.2). Unrecognized and hence untreated causes of acute confusion may also occasionally need to be identified so that appropriate treatment can resolve the confusion. In particular, drug therapy is essential information and should include any over-the-counter medications that may have been purchased.

Table 6.2 *Long-standing confusion—conditions to exclude*

Space-occupying lesion
—tumour: primary or secondary
—subdural haematoma
Normal pressure hydrocephalus
Depression
Drugs—especially alcohol
Myxoedema (occasionally thyrotoxicosis)
Vitamin B_{12}/folate deficiency
Neurosyphilis
Unrecognized (and hence untreated) causes of acute confusion (*see* Table 6.1)

Minimum investigations should include a full blood count, erythrocyte sedimentation rate (ESR) and measurement of serum electrolytes, glucose, calcium and liver enzymes. Thyroid function tests, vitamin B_{12} and folate levels, treponemal serology, a chest X-ray and ECG should also be routinely performed. Visualization of the brain is most readily achieved by CT scanning. Regrettably, this investigation is not yet generally available, but is desirable for all patients with suspected dementia. However, in places where this approach is impractical, CT scanning must be reserved for such patients who are considered likely to have structural lesions, such as cerebral tumours or normal pressure hydrocephalus.

Special clinics, usually euphemistically named 'memory' or 'memory disorders' clinics have been set up in various parts of the country, and are making a small but important impact on the problem of dementia by excluding treatable causes. As well as being places where research is actively pursued, they aim to identify early dementia, where this has been previously undiagnosed, and to coordinate the various supportive services that are available.

Management of dementia

Although there is no specific therapeutic agent with proven efficacy in any form of dementia, much can be done in general terms to support affected patients and their carers. Dementia, more than any other physical illness, threatens sufferers' abilities to organize their day-to-day affairs and live independent lives. Attention to the general health of patients with dementia is of the utmost importance, in order to prevent additional remedial illnesses, such as anaemia, heart failure or vitamin deficiencies, that may further worsen their mental impairment. Specific management of an affected patient falls into two components: the control of any disordered behaviour, and management of the patient in her social environment, usually at home. It is important to support patients in their own homes for as long as possible, provided that neither they, nor those caring for them, suffer unduly. Not only are institutional resources for affected patients scarce, but also patients generally fare better in surroundings that are familiar to them.

Treatment of disordered behaviour

Sedatives and major tranquillizers may be helpful in management of patients with dementia (as well as those with acute confusional states). However, as a general rule, their use should be kept to an absolute minimum, as side-effects are both dangerous and common. If used inappropriately, they may even increase the confusion.

Nocturnal restlessness and wandering are common and may require drug therapy. It is important to determine a patient's pre-morbid sleep pattern and tailor therapy to it. We must not expect everyone to sleep from 11 p.m. to 7 a.m.—some patients may have gone to bed much earlier and others much later for most of their lives. A hypnotic, given just before a patient's normal retiring time, should improve the situation. However, restlessness due to pain or discomfort from constipation or urinary frequency must be treated specifically. A hypnotic with a large safety margin, such as chlormethiazole, is recommended for elderly patients, and this is available in tablet or syrup form. The benzodiazepines and barbiturates cause elderly patients to suffer significant sedation, which is carried over to the following morning. Being drugs of addiction, confusion may also be induced when these drugs are suddenly withdrawn.

Daytime restlessness and agitation may respond to the calming effects of well-ordered, quiet surroundings, together with positive steps to assist orientation, e.g. clocks readily visible to tell the time of day. If these simple measures are unsuccessful, regular treatment with thioridazine (10–50 mg t.d.s.) or haloperidol (0.5–1 mg b.d. or t.d.s.) may be added. Both drugs are useful in having only slight sedative effects, although thioridazine may occasionally be associated with anticholinergic side-effects and haloperidol may cause troublesome extrapyramidal reactions.

Mild paranoid symptoms are common in dementia. When paranoia has been established, thioridazine or trifluoperazine (1–3 mg b.d. or t.d.s.), may be extremely effective in alleviating or abolishing the symptoms. For the rare occurrence of uncontrolled restlessness or aggressive behaviour, parenteral anti-psychotic agents may be given. In such instances, chlorpromazine (25–100 mg) or haloperidol (2–5 mg), given intramuscularly, will be effective and cause rapid sedation. However, both drugs may frequently cause extrapyramidal reactions and tardive dyskinesia, while chlorpromazine may be associated with the development of cholestatic jaundice and also hypotension, due to its anticholinergic effects. Sudden changes in behaviour, however, should always raise the suspicion of the development of an acute confusional state, which may be reversed with appropriate treatment.

Management of the patient's environment

Once behavioural problems have been controlled as far as possible, the question is posed of determining where the patient is able to live—i.e. can she manage or be managed at home, or is institutional care needed? For patients with mild dementia who live alone, the services of a regular home help and daily 'meals on wheels' may provide sufficient assistance at first. Patients who live with their spouses, children or other relatives may be adequately cared for, as long as both patient and carer are physically fit. Problems of care caused by physical disability of the carers can often be overcome by the provision of social services' or district nurse support. Community psychogeriatric nurses (CPNs), where deemed appropriate by the local psychogeriatric service, may help by providing not only continued supervision of the patients and of the administration of their drugs but also counselling and support of the carers. Other measures that may be available include assistance with bathing by the district nurse and the provision of domiciliary chiropody. Where incontinence is an established problem, the provision of disposable incontinence pads or an incontinence laundry service may help.

People who look after relatives with dementia are often bewildered by their behaviour and forgetfulness. Relatives' support groups can give powerful self-help for those facing the common problem of living with a demented relative, a process which has been likened to a living bereavement. Support for such households within the community must be sought and energetically employed. Home helps, paid 'good neighbours', street and estate wardens, and sheltered housing complexes are all means of assisting or replacing family support. Day care at a Day Centre may provide some regular monitoring of patients who live alone or relief for carers, who otherwise provide constant care, day and night. Holiday 'respite' admissions to a local authority residential home or a hospital ward may also provide a vital break for the caring relatives. However, such admissions are not without some risk, as a move to unfamiliar surroundings may lead to a temporary increase in disturbed behaviour.

Institutional care may finally become necessary for a minority of demented elderly people, though, unhappily, reasonable demands for such institutional care far outstrip its supply at the present time. Where patients living alone are unable to maintain an independent existence, even with the full support of social services, and where mobility and continence are preserved with no significant behavioural disturbance, admission to a local authority residential home may be appropriate. With patients whose physical disability requires considerable nursing care, the choice lies, depending upon local circumstances, between nursing-home and long-term hospital care. Psychogeriatric or geriatric hospital care is required when the behaviour of such patients remains disturbed, the choice depending on the degree of physical disability and behavioural disturbance.

OTHER PSYCHIATRIC DISORDERS OF ELDERLY PEOPLE

Depression

Elderly people are as likely to become depressed as those who are younger. Unfortunately the diagnosis is often overlooked, especially where an elderly person may have a serious illness or disability that may be regarded as sufficient to account for the observed unhappiness. Social isolation and the well-documented increased risk of suicide makes the treatment of depression in elderly people important, often with hospital admission being necessary. Hypochondriasis, often with bowel complaints, may mask a hidden depressive illness in a person with an anxious or neurotic personality. Severe depression, with withdrawal and apathy, may be mistaken for dementia (pseudodementia), while many depressed elderly people may hide their depression, putting on a brave face when talking to a doctor.

A careful history and examination can often separate depression from dementia (though the two may also co-exist). Depressed patients tend to be poorly motivated, have a reduced concentration span and often have a past history of depression. They will also make minimal efforts to compensate for any cognitive loss.

Bereavement is a common precipitant of depression, although physical illness is, perhaps, even more important. The development of depression, with its somatic effects on appetite and sleep as well as mood, often follows a stroke, especially in the presence of dysphasia. Unrecognized and untreated, the depression of a patient with a stroke may form a very real barrier to successful rehabilitation. Depression may be the only manifestation of hypothyroidism in elderly patients, which disappears with the regular administration of thyroxine.

Alcoholism and depression may often co-exist and present as an 'acute confusional state', sometimes with wandering or 'failure to cope' at home. (Alcoholism may also be associated with the development of dementia, as well as various nutritional deficiencies (*see* p. 45). Like many iatrogenic conditions, drugs may also cause depression. Methyl dopa, occasionally still used in the treatment of hypertension, is commonly implicated.

Treatment with antidepressant agents is usually successful, though electroconvulsant therapy may have a valuable place in selected, severely affected patients. The tricyclic antidepressant drugs are the most effective agents, but care is needed to adjust the dosage in elderly patients to obtain the maximum benefit, with the minimum of anticholinergic side-effects.

Paraphrenia

Paraphrenia is an uncommon form of schizophrenia, occurring for the first time late in life. It takes the form of a paranoid psychosis, which is restricted in form and content, frequently with paranoid delusions about one or several neighbours, with resultant noisy abuse directed towards them. Consequent allegations, when mild, may often be difficult to differentiate from the normal suspicions and fears of an elderly person living alone. Auditory hallucinations may be present, often in patients who are sensorily impaired. However, this condition tends to occur in people who have led isolated and withdrawn lives and may be related to their previous personalities. It is often simply treated with phenothiazines, of which trifluperazine and thioridazine have the least troublesome side-effects.

Diogenes syndrome

The Diogenes syndrome describes a rare form of personality disorder, where an elderly person is found living in a state of extreme neglect and squalor, frequently with an exaggerated tendency to hoard rubbish. When brought to the attention of the medical profession, either because of complaints by neighbours or during a physical illness, such people are usually found to be of sound mind, of moderate financial means and tending to come from an affluent socio-economic background. The condition is not so much a syndrome, as the end-stage of a life-long personality disorder. Interference with this life-style should only be attempted if harm is likely to be caused to the person concerned or to neighbours, e.g. by causing a public health hazard. By the time such people come to the attention of the medical profession, they may have several physical disorders that need treatment. Rehabilitation of such people has been said to be possible.

LEGAL ASPECTS OF MENTAL DISORDER

Elderly people have the same rights and duties in law as any other group of citizens. Mental and physical illness may pose difficulties for elderly people in exercising their rights; in certain circumstances, others may act on their behalf and may, in extreme cases governed by Acts of Parliament, even override their wishes.

Court of Protection

In the UK, the Court of Protection exists to safeguard the interests of any person who, because of mental incapacity, cannot manage his or her own affairs. It is an office of the Lord Chancellor's Department, but also a Court of Law, with a Master, an assistant Master and other officers, nominated by the Lord Chancellor. The Court takes over responsibility for the financial affairs of the patient (but this is only applicable if there are substantial assets). The majority of people under the Court's protection are elderly.

Application can be made by anyone, but is most often made by a social worker, directly to the Court (The Court of Protection, Store Street, London, WC1E 7BP) or indirectly via a solicitor, and an Originating Application form is completed. The doctor in charge of the patient is required to complete a medical certificate (form CP3) about the medical reasons why the patient is believed incapable of managing her own affairs. In addition, other personal details need to be given, such as how far the patient can appreciate her surroundings, how often she receives visitors and the likely prognosis of her mental disability. If completion of this certificate (CP3) proves difficult, it may be helpful to seek the advice of a psychiatrist.

The name of a person who will act on the patient's behalf, called the Receiver, is put forward. This person is usually the nearest relative but can be any other relative or friend, or a solicitor. The papers are examined by the Court and, if satisfactory, the patient is served with a *Notice of Originating Proceedings*. If the patient is incapable of managing her own affairs, she may well be unable to understand the implications of this Notice. Another form must then be completed, to provide proof that an explanation has been given to the patient as to what has been proposed. Following this, the patient has a legal right to object (in writing) within seven days, either directly or via a solicitor. If there is no objection, the proceedings continue and a Receiver is appointed. The Court oversees the management of the estate and requires the Receiver to account, usually every year, for his or her dealings.

Power of attorney

The power of attorney is a simpler arrangement by which any person, e.g. a hospital patient (called the donor), gives authority to another (the attorney) to act, on limited or generalized matters, on his or her behalf. Such actions are to be based on the wishes of the donor. A legal document, drawn up by a lawyer, is signed in the presence of a witness to show that the attorney has power to act on the donor's behalf. It may be shown to banks, pension funds, insurance companies, etc. However, it cannot validly be given if the donor suffers mental incapacity, such that this arrangement cannot be appreciated, or she cannot make her wishes known, for example, due to dysphasia after a stroke. It ceases to be valid if mental incapacity later develops (when Court of Protection (*see* above) must be sought).

Such a situation can now be overcome with an application of an Enduring Power of Attorney (EPA), whereby such powers may continue after the donor becomes mentally incapable. This allows a simpler procedure of changing from the set of circumstances where the donor is mentally sound to that where a Court of Protection order applies, when the donor becomes mentally impaired. Both donor and attorney need fully to understand the nature of the EPA at the outset. If the attorney believes the donor is, or is becoming, mentally incapable, the Court of Protection must be notified so that the affairs and property of that person can be managed for their benefit, with the records and account of such dealings duly monitored.

Compulsory care

Section 47, National Assistance Act, 1948

Section 47 of the 1948 *National Assistance Act* gave the Medical Officer of Health the power to apply to a magistrate for the compulsory removal of persons who:

(a) are suffering from grave chronic illness, or being aged infirm or physically incapacitated, are living in insanitary conditions and
(b) are unable to devote to themselves, and are not receiving from other persons, proper care and attention.

It also gave the Medical Officer of Health powers to remove a person to prevent 'injury to the health of or serious nuisance to other persons'.

[In the 1974 reorganization of the NHS, Medical Officers of Health have been replaced by Community Physicians (recently renamed Consultants in Public Health Medicine). In health authorities without health districts, the Medical Officer for Environmental Health is responsible for operating this section; in health authorities with health districts, the District Director of Public Health is responsible.] To obtain an order for removal, he had to give seven days notice (to allow the person concerned the right of appeal) to a Court of Summary Jurisdiction. If the Court agreed, the person could be 'detained' for up to three months in a 'suitable hospital or other place'. However, the necessary seven days delay in such circumstances could have serious consequences for the person concerned, perhaps allowing death, which the order may have been trying to prevent. However, in 1951, an amendment was introduced by a back-bench MP, Doctor later Sir Alfred Broughton, which allowed the removal without delay for a period of three weeks, provided that the Medical Officer of Health's opinion was supported by that of another registered medical practitioner.

Although there are no national statistics kept of the use of Section 47, it has been estimated that it is used about 200 times each year throughout England, in the vast majority of cases involving people over 65 years of age. The powers encompassed by Section 47 cannot be used lightly, as they infringe the liberty of people living in the manner of their choice. However, there will always be a small number of elderly people who require hospital admission, but who refuse it, although they are not mentally disordered, do not want to die and wish to get better. Reasons for this attitude are many and may include fear of permanent institutionalization and fear of the 'workhouse', which many geriatric hospitals are still considered to be. Perhaps the commonest reason is the mistaken belief of many elderly people that all their problems are untreatable because of their age and must therefore be accepted rather than treated. Although at present there is no legal requirement for a specialist geriatric opinion, the geriatrician is particularly well-trained to assess this type of situation and, more often than not, is involved in the use of these powers.

Mental Health Act, 1983

Patients who have a mental illness, such that they are considered a danger to themselves or others, may similarly be compulsorily admitted to hospital for assessment and/or treatment of the mental condition. Such action invokes the *Mental Health Act* 1983, with different sections having varying medical requirements, rights of appeal and durations of compulsory admission. Doctors who may be approved to invoke this Act are usually Consultant Psychiatrists, under whose care the patient is subsequently admitted, and the patient's general practitioner. Geriatricians need to know about this procedure, though they are hardly ever involved in these cases.

Conclusions

Legal powers, such as have been outlined above, pose some fundamental questions which society as a whole needs to address. Care of sick elderly people (whether mentally or physically ill) still occasionally verges on the patronizing, paternalistic and over-protective. Answers currently vary widely to questions such as: 'How far should old people be allowed to live in squalor if they refuse help?'; 'How to balance the risks of hospitalization and institutionalization against the risks of remaining independent?'; and 'How can the legal and social rights of mentally disabled old people be protected?' Such questions need a more satisfactory solution than at present.

Chapter

7

Common Forms of Cerebrovascular Disease

STROKE • TRANSIENT ISCHAEMIC ATTACKS • TEMPORAL ARTERITIS

STROKE

Strokes caused by cerebrovascular disease are a major cause of disability in the elderly population and form the third commonest cause of death in the Western world, after heart disease and cancer. The incidence of stroke rises steeply with age; two-thirds of all strokes occur in people over the age of 70, men and women being affected equally. Stroke is defined as an acute disturbance of cerebral function of presumed vascular origin, with disability lasting more than 24 hours, which may be due to either:

1. A thrombotic/embolic occlusion of a cerebral artery, producing infarction (approximately 85% of cases).
2. Less commonly, to a spontaneous rupture of a vessel, producing an intracerebral or subarachnoid haemorrhage (approx. 15% of cases).

If the focal neurological deficit resolves completely within 24 hours, it is called a transient ischaemic attack (TIA), *see* p. 72.

The cerebral circulation

Although it comprises only 2% of the total body weight, the brain uses about 20% of the total body oxygen consumption. In addition, it also requires a plentiful supply of glucose and other nutrients. After any injury, neural tissue is incapable of cell division or regeneration. The brain is therefore critically dependent on its blood supply. The circulation of blood to the brain is derived from the two internal carotid arteries and two vertebral arteries, which arise from the major arteries in the neck and which subdivide within the skull, anastomosing at the base of the brain to form the circle of Willis. This anastomosis functions to protect the brain from damage caused by partial occlusion within the major vessels. However, major disruptions of blood flow cannot be accommodated without the occurrence of cerebral damage. Autoregulatory mechanisms within the cerebral vasculature also serve to protect the cerebral circulation from variations in perfusion arising from the heart. Cerebral blood flow declines progressively with increasing age, while the autoregulatory mechanisms, which normally require a mean systolic arterial pressure of 80–90 mmHg, may become impaired in the presence of vascular disease.

Causes of stroke (Table 7.1)

The major underlying pathological process in the aetiology of stroke is the formation of *atheroma* within the walls of the cerebral arteries. Atheromatous plaques narrow the lumen of the arteries while the overlying endothelial lining may become ulcerated, stimulating thrombosis or the formation of emboli, which will subsequently lodge in smaller vessels of the brain. The areas within the vessels that are particularly prone to atheroma formation are those where there is greatest turbulence: at the origin of the great vessels on the aortic arch, the bifurcation of the common carotids and, within the circle of Willis, at the points of division within the middle cerebral arteries.

The formation of atheroma is accelerated in the presence of systemic hypertension and diabetes mellitus. Hypertension is a well-recognized risk factor in the incidence of stroke, causing not only cerebral infarction, but also haemorrhage. It is associated not only with atheroma but with the formation and rupture of micro-aneurysms on vessels deep within the brain substance. Atheroma is a generalized phenomenon, affecting blood vessels throughout the body, including the coronary arteries. A stroke may follow the development of a myocardial infarction, due to coronary artery atheroma, having been caused by embolization from a mural thrombus that formed overlying the infarcted tissue. There are numerous other sources of emboli that may arise within the heart, e.g. a thrombus in the left atrium due to

Table 7.1 *Causes of stroke*

Conditions affecting blood vessels—producing vessel occlusion or platelet emboli	Atheroma (hypertension, diabetes mellitus) Arteritis (polyarteritis nodosa, systemic lupus arteritis, syphilis)
Haemodynamic disturbances	Hypertension Hypotension (e.g. after myocardial infarct, pulmonary embolus, gastrointestinal haemorrhage)
Sources of emboli within the heart	Atrial fibrillation, atrial myxoma Mural thrombus after myocardial infarct Endocarditis (rheumatic heart disease, bacterial endocarditis) Prosthetic cardiac valves
Conditions altering blood constituents	Cellular components (e.g. polycythaemia, leukaemia, thrombocytosis) Hyperviscosity syndromes affecting plasma proteins
Drugs	e.g. Antihypertensive agents

atrial fibrillation and mitral stenosis or emboli from diseased heart valves themselves.

As well as hypertension being implicated, any episode of *hypo*tension may equally cause cerebral infarction, whether following a myocardial infarct, pulmonary embolus or gastrointestinal bleed, because of failure of the autoregulatory mechanisms to maintain cerebral perfusion. Elderly people are very susceptible to potent antihypertensive therapy, so that hypotension may be produced and itself induce a stroke, rather than the original hypertension being treated. Rarer causes of stroke include conditions where arteritis occurs or where the viscosity of blood is increased from excess circulating cells or proteins.

Differential diagnosis

Most patients with a sudden onset of focal neurological signs will have cerebrovascular disease. However, a minority of patients with other conditions masquerading as a stroke need to be identified, especially as many may successfully be treated and returned to normal life again (Table 7.2). The most dramatic group are diabetic patients with hypoglycaemia, perhaps because of excess insulin or the prolonged action of many of the oral hypoglycaemic agents. Such patients may occasionally present with focal neurological signs, which are completely reversed by the administration of glucose. However, if the diagnosis is delayed and hypoglycaemia allowed to persist, permanent cerebral damage may occur.

Table 7.2 *Differential diagnosis of stroke—conditions to exclude*

Hypoglycaemia
Cerebral tumour—benign
—malignant
Subdural haematoma
Migraine
Epilepsy
Infection—intracerebral abscess
—meningitis

Elderly patients with space-occupying lesions only rarely present with headache, vomiting and papilloedema, typically indicative of raised intracranial pressure. A history of a head injury is often absent, but there is frequently a slowly progressive deterioration of neurological function (over months) and, in the presence of focal signs, both should raise the suspicion of a slowly expanding blood clot or tumour.

Computerized tomography (CT) of the head is the diagnostic investigation of choice. Evacuation of a subdural haematoma or the removal of a benign cerebral tumour will frequently cause dramatic improvement. The diagnosis of a malignant cerebral tumour mimicking a stroke is important to prevent inappropriate rehabilitation being undertaken.

Hemiplegia may occasionally follow an epileptic fit (Todd's paralysis), or be associated with a migraine attack, which will show rapid and complete spontaneous recovery. However, an epileptic fit may arise coincidentally in a patient who has had a stroke, both being caused by the same underlying cerebrovascular disease.

A stroke may be associated with meningism, i.e. neck stiffness and fever, if a small quantity of blood enters the subarachnoid space. It needs to be distinguished carefully from meningitis (which requires a diagnostic lumbar puncture) and from a cerebral abscess, especially in patients with chronic sepsis, such as chronic ear infections or bronchiectasis. Specialist advice needs to be sought for further neurological and bacteriological investigation.

Clinical features

The neurological deficits seen in stroke patients depend upon the area of brain affected. Patients typically present with a sudden onset of weakness (hemiparesis) or paralysis (hemiplegia) of one side of the body and ipsilateral sensory loss. There may be impairment of consciousness initially and absent tendon reflexes because of neurogenic shock, the reflexes later becoming brisker on the affected side, with an associated extensor plantar response. Detailed correlations of neurological deficits and the arterial territories involved will be found in specialist neurological texts. However, it is important to examine stroke patients as fully as possible to assess all the neurological deficits, besides the obvious motor and sensory loss, as such deficits will need to be appreciated by everyone in the rehabilitation team before optimal treatment can be planned.

Assessment of communication

If the patient is conscious, assessment of communication is a vital first step. Deafness should be identified, if present, and ear wax removed or a portable speech amplifier employed as necessary. Patients may be *dysarthric* and not able to speak clearly if tongue and facial muscles are affected. *Aphasia* occurs when the dominant hemisphere is affected and is traditionally of two types: receptive or sensory aphasia is the term used to describe difficulty in understanding what is said, while expressive or motor dysphasia describes problems in formulating words and planning movements necessary for speaking. Other classifications of aphasia use the fluency of verbal expression—non-fluent aphasia being used to describe patients who speak slowly and with difficulty, producing few words, whereas patients with fluent aphasia are those who speak freely and without effort, but the speech they produce is without meaning because the words and grammar used are incorrect. Global aphasia describes the disability of patients who can understand little or no speech and are able to utter only a few sounds.

At the same time as speech is considered, it is often helpful to assess the adequacy of patients' *swallowing*. Dehydration is common initially, because of inadequate fluid intake, and intravenous fluids may be necessary as a temporary measure before enteral feeding can be re-established. Speech therapists may often be able to give assistance to promote the return of normal swallowing mechanisms.

Balance and proprioception

Proprioception or joint-position sense arises in muscles, tendons, ligaments and joints and is conveyed to the parietal lobes by the posterior columns of the spinal cord. However, if joint-position sense is lost because of damage to these pathways, coordination of movement will be impaired. (NB. weakness of a limb will automatically produce poor muscle coordination in that limb.) With midline brain stem and cerebellar lesions, truncal ataxia may be produced, so that patients are unable to sit unsupported as their perceived centre of gravity is outside their body and they slump to one side, or if attempting to stand, they lean to one side and fall over.

Perception

Perception is the ability to interpret sensation—sensation of any modality, e.g. tactile, visual or auditory. Disorders of perception are common and often overlooked by the medical staff who may become frustrated by stroke patients' apparent lack of improvement after what is seen as good return of motor power. Such patients may be labelled as 'not trying' or just 'awkward'. The parietal lobes are concerned with spatial and discriminative aspects of sensation. If damaged, two clinical signs may be found: sensory inattention and agnosia.

Sensory inattention to, for example, tactile stimuli may be demonstrated by touching both hands of a patient simultaneously. In the presence of normal sensation in both hands when tested individually, sensation arising from the affected hand is ignored when both are touched at the same time.

Agnosia is the term used to denote the inability to interpret sensory stimuli. For example, tactile agnosia is the inability to recognize the form and shape of an object, e.g. a coin, placed in the hand (also called astereognosis). However, appreciation of space and body image is also important for full recovery from a stroke. Spatial agnosia or neglect occurs particularly in patients with damaged non-dominant parietal lobes and may manifest itself by them ignoring one side of their environment, e.g. they may finish their meal and yet be unaware that food has been left on one side of the plate. Problems of body image may be disturbing for the patient as well as the medical staff. Self agnosia may result in a lack of awareness of a part of the body or failure to recognize its disability. A hemiplegic patient may not appreciate that one arm is weak or that she cannot walk and, in such cases, her cooperation with rehabilitation becomes extremely difficult. Visuo-spatial sense may be impaired, with patients being unable to find their way around in their own home or in the hospital ward. Failure to differentiate right from left may also become apparent.

Apraxia

Apraxia is the motor counterpart of agnosia and is the inability to perform skilled movement patterns in the absence of motor weakness or sensory loss. Apraxia and agnosia are closely linked parietal lobe functions and perceptual tests cannot readily distinguish between them. The normal sequence of movements involved in say, filling a kettle with water or dressing, may be quite impossible for a patient, even though comprehension, muscle power, sensation and coordination are adequate. Recognition of these difficulties may direct therapy in the appropriate direction, for example, practice with sequencing of actions. If full recovery is impossible, dressing, for example, may become possible only if clothes are arranged in the order they are put on.

Vision

The two main deficits to look for are visual field defects, where there is complete loss of vision of half (or less) of each visual field, and visual inattention or neglect of one half of vision. In the initial phase of rehabilitation, it is important to have objects such as cups or spectacles on a hospital locker visible on the unaffected side. Later, with patients who have visual neglect, these objects can be situated on the affected side to encourage them to reach over the mid-line to that side. Rarely the visual cortex of the occipital cortex is affected bilaterally by a stroke, and cortical blindness of both eyes results.

Treatment of stroke

The initial treatment of stroke patients is that directed towards the care of any patient with impaired mobility and communication—checking hydration (looking for any swallowing difficulties), skin care, and attending to bladder and bowel function.

Physiotherapy

Physiotherapy is important to regain muscle strength and coordination. Even if consciousness is impaired initially and voluntary movement absent, passive movements of limbs will keep joints freely mobile and may reduce the development of spasticity later. If an arm is sufficiently weak, the stability of the shoulder joint, which predominantly arises from the surrounding muscles, is compromised and painful subluxation may occur. This may be prevented by correct positioning of the arm, but the assistance of a shoulder support may be needed for a time. Pneumonia and pulmonary emboli are frequent complications following a stroke. Their treatment is the same as for any younger patient.

Rehabilitation

After a stroke, rehabilitation centres around the paramedical staff: the physiotherapist, occupational therapist and, where appropriate, the speech therapist. It is essential that stroke patients are fully assessed to detect their less obvious neurological deficits and that this information is passed on to all those who come into contact with them. In particular, the nursing staff on the ward need to be aware of visual problems, any sensory inattention or other perceptual difficulties for optimum treatment of these patients.

Treatment of hypertension

Although hypertension is a well-known risk factor in stroke, blood pressure is often found to be raised initially as a direct consequence of the stroke but will fall spontaneously to pre-stroke levels within a couple of weeks. Unless extreme levels are recorded, antihypertensive drugs should not be used, at least initially. Rapid lowering of blood pressure may worsen brain ischaemia even further.

Other drug therapy

For patients who have had a cerebral embolus, secondary to atrial fibrillation and the breaking up of a clot in the left atrium or to a mural thrombus in the heart, anticoagulation may offer an effective means of preventing a recurrence. However, before embarking upon anticoagulation, it is essential to exclude the presence of a cerebral haemorrhage, as such treatment will worsen the cerebral damage already present. CT scanning of the head is the only reliable means of distinguishing cerebral haemorrhage from infarction and should always be undertaken before anticoagulation is considered.

A number of drugs have been proposed to limit the neurological damage caused by a stroke by reducing the cerebral oedema initially present or by improving cerebral perfusion to ischaemic areas. High dose steroids, intravenous glycerol and various vasodilators have all been used, but without consistent benefit; their use is not recommended.

Psychological effects of stroke

In addition to attending to the underlying causes of strokes and their physical sequelae, it is of great importance to remember the psychological impact of the disease on the patient and family. A reaction akin to bereavement is often felt by both patient and family about the 'loss' sustained. This may be manifest by poor motivation during rehabilitation. Depression following upon the realization of residual disability is common after a stroke and requires sensitive handling. The place of antidepressant medication is poorly documented. Emotional lability, i.e. excessive and inappropriate weepiness or (less commonly) laughter, may occur; this may be distressing for patients and family alike. It should not be confused with the psychological sequelae of a stroke as it reflects specific neurological damage to the frontal lobes or upper brain stem.

Prognosis

Stroke carries a high mortality; 50% of patients die in the first two weeks after the acute event. However, in those who survive, some recovery will occur, depending upon the extent of the cerebral damage. Impaired consciousness at presentation is the most important adverse prognostic sign in terms of mortality and functional recovery. Various authors have described the functional outcome after the first two to four weeks. Most agree that about a third of patients return home and resume their normal activities, some 10% of these having no neurological deficit. A further third are limited to some extent, but are able to go home if well-supported by family or friends. Only a third of patients remain severely disabled and require continued nursing care.

As the majority of stroke patients have widespread vascular disease, they are at increased risk, not only of further strokes, but also of developing the manifestations of cardiac atheroma. A patient who has recovered from a stroke is more likely to die from a myocardial infarction than from developing another stroke.

Prevention of stroke

The control of hypertension in all age groups is well-established as a means of reducing the incidence of stroke. Prevention of polycythaemia in susceptible subjects by repeated venesection will improve blood viscosity, as will treatment of other haematological disorders associated with an increased blood viscosity. Anticoagulation after a cerebral embolus (especially in patients with mitral stenosis and atrial fibrillation) is a reasonable treatment option, although there is controversy about the timing of such treatment—whether to start immediately or after an interval of one to two weeks, in order to decrease the risk of haemorrhage within the infarct.

Platelet aggregation is now thought to contribute to arterial thrombosis and hence to embolism, ischaemia and infarction, particularly in the cerebral circulation. Platelet aggregation and embolization are thought to arise at sites of atherosclerotic damage within the circulation. In the presence of atherosclerotic disease within the external carotid arteries and intracranial vessels, drugs that prevent platelet aggregation may reduce the incidence of stroke. Controlled trials have demonstrated that aspirin, having powerful in vitro antiplatelet properties, has a small beneficial effect in the prevention of further cerebral damage in patients who have already had strokes or transient ischaemic attacks.

TRANSIENT ISCHAEMIC ATTACKS

A transient (cerebral) ischaemic attack (TIA) is defined as an episode of focal loss of neurological function in which full recovery occurs within

24 hours. TIAs may cause focal signs in the carotid or vertebrobasilar artery territories (Table 7.3). Occasionally they may be heralded by loss of consciousness. Transient monocular blindness (amaurosis fugax) is caused by embolization in the retinal circulation. The emboli may be composed of clumps of platelets or fragments of atheroma. Vision is usually restored to normal within 20 minutes and, in many cases, no permanent cerebral or retinal symptoms subsequently occur.

Table 7.3 *Common symptoms of TIAs*

Carotid territory	*Vertebrobasilar territory*
Monoparesis or hemiparesis	Weakness in any combination of four limbs
Paraesthesia or anaesthesia	Perioral paraesthesia and facial weakness
Speech disorder—predominantly dysphasia	Speech disorder—predominantly dysarthria
Monocular loss of vision (amaurosis fugax)	Diplopia
	Ataxia, vertigo and nystagmus
	Alterations of consciousness

TIAs share the same causes as completed strokes, but are usually due to emboli arising from the atheromatous lining of one or more of the four major arteries supplying the brain. They need to be distinguished carefully from migraine and epilepsy. The importance of TIAs lies in the fact that a third of patients who have one (especially in the carotid territory), go on to develop a completed stroke and in a quarter of these, the interval is less than a month. Therefore, investigations should be directed towards treating predisposing factors, e.g. hypertension, cardiac or haematological conditions, to prevent the occurrence of a subsequent stroke.

As mentioned above, there is some evidence that high-dose aspirin and other drugs affecting platelet aggregation may, in patients who have had a TIA, reduce the incidence of subsequent strokes.

The presence of a carotid bruit in a fit person who has had a carotid TIA raises the possibility of considering angiography to determine if there is a surgically correctable lesion. However, angiography and subsequent arterial surgery are controversial areas of medical practice, not without risk, and are therefore hardly ever considered in the treatment of elderly patients.

TEMPORAL ARTERITIS

Temporal arteritis (giant cell arteritis) is an arteritis of medium-sized vessels in which the arterial walls become thickened by granulomatous tissue that contains numerous giant cells and a chronic inflammatory infiltrate. An important consequence of the arteritis is the frequent segmental occlusion of the affected vessels by thrombosis and intimal proliferation.

The incidence of temporal arteritis rises with increasing age, the elderly being commonly affected. The diagnosis needs to be made and treatment initiated promptly, because if the retinal arteries are involved and the condition untreated, there is the risk of visual impairment or blindness. Cerebral vessels are occasionally affected and may produce a stroke. However, the temporal arteries are most commonly affected and, in the acute phase, become tender, hot and thickened. Patients may complain of temporal headache, while there may also be systemic symptoms of fever, weight loss, malaise or generalized aches and pains.

The diagnosis is suggested by the history and a high erythrocyte sedimentation rate (ESR); it is confirmed, if possible, by biopsy of an affected artery. Prednisolone, at an initial high dose (40–60 mg daily), will produce a dramatic improvement in symptoms and cause the ESR to fall. It can then be reduced to 10–20 mg daily within two weeks and maintained around 10–15 mg daily for the next year, before tailing off to zero is attempted.

Polymyalgia rheumatica

Temporal arteritis is similar to another condition, *polymyalgia rheumatica*, also found commonly in older people. It is associated with temporal arteritis in 15% of cases. Typically it causes pain and stiffness in proximal muscles, especially of the upper limbs, and may cause systemic symptoms of fever, malaise, and anaemia of the normochromic, normocytic type. There are no focal arterial lesions. The diagnosis is suggested by the history. The ESR is typically high, and prednisolone, as for temporal arteritis, produces rapid relief of symptoms and normalization of the ESR. Because of the well-known side-effects of corticosteroid therapy, the dose of prednisolone is reduced as quickly as possible while maintaining its maximal therapeutic benefit.

Chapter

8

Common Diseases of the Nervous System

PARKINSONISM • NEUROLOGICAL PROBLEMS DUE TO IMPAIRED AUTONOMIC FUNCTION • NORMAL PRESSURE HYDROCEPHALUS • CHRONIC SUBDURAL HAEMATOMA • CERVICAL SPONDYLOSIS • EPILEPSY

PARKINSONISM

Parkinsonism is a common disease of elderly people. It differs slightly from the classical Parkinson's disease that affects people in middle age, as first described by Sir James Parkinson, by the relative lack of tremor and the tendency to dementia. It is a chronic and progressive condition associated with a three-fold increase in mortality, compared with a population of the same age and sex. The underlying common histological feature is a deficiency of the neurotransmitter, dopamine, in the pigmented nuclei of the brain stem.

Types of Parkinsonism (Table 8.1)

Several forms of Parkinsonism are recognized other than the classical, idiopathic type. Many young patients developed a *slowly progressive type* of Parkinsonism following the pandemic of encephalitis lethargica, which occurred during the period 1918 to 1926. They demonstrated several specific features, such as oculogyric crises, in addition to the other well-recognized features of Parkinsonism. Most sufferers from this form of Parkinsonism have now died and no other cohort of post-infective patients has been recognized.

Drug-induced Parkinsonism is regrettably common and can result

Table 8.1 *Types of Parkinsonism*

Idiopathic
Post-encephalitic
Drug-induced
Secondary Parkinsonism, e.g. associated with Huntington's chorea, Shy-Drager syndrome
('Arteriosclerotic')

from treatment with any neuroleptic drug with dopamine-receptor blocking activity. Causative drugs commonly overlooked are metochlopramide (Maxolon), prochlorperazine (Stemetil) and various antidepressant–anxiolytic–neuroleptic combinations (such as Motival). Drug withdrawal will usually produce recovery within six months, but occasionally up to two years is needed.

Of considerable theoretical interest is the recently described pure (and L-dopa responsive) Parkinsonism resulting from the deliberate self-administration of, or occupational exposure to, the mepiridine analogue 1-methyl-4-phenyl-1,2,3,6-tetrahydropyridine (MPTP), which appears to be readily metabolized to become a specific toxin to dopaminergic neurones in the basal ganglia.

Features of Parkinsonism may be found in the presence of *other chronic neurological disorders*, such as Huntington's chorea, Wilson's disease and progressive supranuclear palsy.

A form of Parkinsonism, so-called *arteriosclerotic Parkinsonism*, has until recently been thought to be associated with cerebral arteriosclerosis, occurring in elderly, hypertensive patients with evidence of dementia. This term was used to describe the akinesia of multi-infarct cerebral disease (*see* p. 51). Brain histology and computerized tomography (CT) scan do not substantiate this aetiology, though both conditions may occur coincidentally. Hence this is no longer considered to be a true form of Parkinsonism and indeed such patients are rarely helped by anti-Parkinsonism therapy.

Histological and biochemical features

Histological examination of the brains of patients with Parkinsonism and classical Parkinson's disease demonstrates the destruction and loss of pigmented melanin-bearing neurones in the basal ganglia, especially the substantia nigra, locus coeruleus and also the dorsal motor nucleus of the vagus. These areas contain pathways using the neurotransmitter dopamine. It has been found that symptoms of Parkinsonism develop only after approximately 80% of dopamine receptors have been lost. At the same time as dopamine production is reduced, the normal balance between the dopaminergic and cholinergic pathways is upset, with cholinergic effects being accentuated. Drug treatment is therefore directed towards restoring this balance, by restoring levels of dopamine or reducing those of acetylcholine in the brain.

Clinical features (Table 8.2)

Features of Parkinsonism begin insidiously with the characteristic hand tremor or the general 'slowing down' of hypokinesia, often mistaken for part of the natural ageing process.

Table 8.2 *Clinical features of Parkinsonism*

Hypokinesia/bradykinesia
Rigidity
Tremor
Postural abnormality
Mental disturbance

Tremor of the hand is often extremely embarrassing socially. It may start in one hand, commonly followed by involvement of the lower limb of the same side, before the other hand is involved. It is typically a resting tremor (rate of 4–5 Hz), diminishing on movement and absent during sleep. The tremor is depressed by muscular rigidity and is absent in drug-induced Parkinsonism.

Hypokinesia or poverty of movement may be marked and not necessarily always attributable to muscular rigidity. Initiation or change of movement is difficult and slow. Even in bed, movements such as turning over become increasingly difficult. Associated movements are often absent, e.g. swinging of the arms whilst walking is lost.

Muscular rigidity, affecting agonist and antagonist muscle groups equally, is frequently severe. This gives rise to 'lead pipe' rigidity or, in the presence of a marked tremor, a 'cogwheel' type of rigidity. Fine finger movements are poor and micrographia is an early feature. Speech becomes soft and indistinct and there is difficulty in initiating speech, as the muscles of phonation become involved.

The characteristic *posture* and *gait* is a summation of the effects of muscular rigidity and hypokinesia. Muscular rigidity appears early in the neck with resulting neck flexion. The posture becomes stooping with a pronounced dorsal kyphosis, while the limbs become adducted and flexed. Steps are short and the gait hesitant and shuffling ('festinant'). Control of posture is impaired with a tendency to overbalance and fall. Postural hypotension also contributes to the frequent falls (*see* p. 100).

Facial immobility is usually pronounced, with patients typically having a staring, mask-like face, and is also a consequence of muscular rigidity and hypokinesia. There is a reduction in the frequency of blinking as well as diminished eye movements. Rigidity of the neck muscles keeps the head quite still. The palpebral fissures are widened. Automatic swallowing of saliva may be impaired; dysphagia due to neuromuscular incoordination may be pronounced with severe disability.

It is hardly surprising that *depression* and *irritability* are common. *Dementia* occurs as the disease progresses in at least a quarter of patients. Dementia was not part of the original description of the disease and much debate continues about whether it should be included as a late manifestation of the disease or a frequent coincidental association.

Treatment

General measures

Physiotherapy has much to contribute in improving the mobility of affected patients by helping to overcome the abnormal gait pattern and, with drug therapy, to improve bradykinesia. As patients' mobility becomes increasingly impaired, they and their families frequently become socially isolated and lonely. An organization concerned specifically with this disability, the Parkinson's Disease Society, is often helpful in providing support and practical advice for both patients and their families.

Any intercurrent illness may be particularly hazardous if it interferes with physical activity, even for a short while. The previous level of mobility may be hard to regain, while bradykinesia may cause the rapid development of pressure sores.

Drug therapy

Dopamine itself does not cross the blood–brain barrier but its precursor, *L-dopa*, readily does. L-dopa remains the most effective agent in the treatment of Parkinsonism. It is orally active and generally used in combination with a peripheral dopa decarboxylase inhibitor to prevent degradation before it reaches the brain. L-dopa may be combined with carbidopa in the ratio of 10:1 or 4:1 in Sinemet preparations, or with benzerazide in the ratio of 4:1 in Madopar preparations. Side-effects of nausea and vomiting may occasionally occur, but more distressing is the occurrence of involuntary dyskinetic (i.e. bizarre) movements—myotonic jerks and athetoid movements. These are dose-related and hence dose reduction may be necessary to abolish them. However, at the same time, the therapeutic effects are similarly reduced. With high doses of L-dopa for several years, on-off effects (i.e. rapid, intermittent dyskinesia) and end-of-dose deterioration occur. These are sometimes overcome for a while by more frequent administration of smaller doses of L-dopa. Transient mental confusion and depression may also occur due to the central actions of dopamine.

The *anticholinergic drugs* formed the basis for the treatment of Parkinsonism for many years before L-dopa was found to be more effective and are therefore seldom used now. They produced a modest reduction in rigidity and slight improvement in tremor, but had no effect on bradykinesia. As atropine-like drugs, their side-effects included blurred vision, a dry mouth, urinary retention, constipation and postural hypotension. Confusion was often produced in the very elderly, especially in those patients with pre-existing dementia. This group of drugs may still be useful sometimes for drug-induced Parkinsonism, where it is not possible to withdraw the inducing drugs.

Deprenyl, a monoamine oxidase inhibitor, inhibits the degradation of dopamine and is occasionally useful in potentiating the antikinetic effects of L-dopa. *Bromocriptine*, a dopaminergic ergot derivative, also potentiates the effect of L-dopa, and may allow its dose reduction. However, this beneficial effect may only be for a few months. *Amanti-*

dine, developed as an antiviral drug, has modest anti-Parkinsonian effects in some patients, though tolerance develops after a few months.

BENIGN ESSENTIAL TREMOR

This condition may occasionally occur as part of ageing, without evidence of other neurological disease. The hands are chiefly affected but rhythmic oscillations of the head may also be present. Its prevalence increases with increasing age and studies have shown it to have an inherited basis. Typically, it is relieved by alcohol and β-blockers but exacerbated by β-agonist drugs.

NEUROLOGICAL PROBLEMS DUE TO IMPAIRED AUTONOMIC FUNCTION

Impaired autonomic function occurs with increasing frequency with advancing age (Table 8.3). This may be a direct result of the ageing process or associated with pathological degeneration of the autonomic nervous system. Autonomic dysfunction may be present alone in younger patients with the Shy–Drager syndrome, a rare form of autonomic neuropathy and Parkinsonism, or in older patients as part of the clinical manifestations of other diseases such as diabetes and Parkinsonism. Orthostatic hypotension will be described in Chapter 10.

Table 8.3 *Main clinical features of impaired autonomic function*

Impaired thermoregulation
Orthostatic hypotension
Disordered bowel motility
Incontinence of urine

The autonomic nervous system is intimately involved with the control of gastrointestinal function. Some degree of oesophageal dysfunction is common in the elderly and takes the form of disorganization of the normal swallowing mechanism. This may be seen during a barium swallow radiograph, where a 'corkscrew' appearance to the barium is seen as it passes more slowly than normal down the oesophagus. A similar motor dysfunction may occur in the large bowel, causing gross dilatation of the colon and intractable constipation, though it may be difficult to distinguish this from the effects of life-long constipation or laxative abuse. Diabetic patients with autonomic dysfunction may, alternatively, suffer diarrhoea without evidence of any other gastrointestinal pathology. They may also have impotence and impaired bladder control (*see* p. 140). Impaired thermo-regulation is chiefly of importance in causing accidental hypothermia and will be described more fully here.

Hypothermia

Hypothermia is defined by a core body temperature of 35°C or less. The term accidental hypothermia is used to distinguish it from hypothermia induced for therapeutic reasons.

Measurement of oral temperature is unreliable if hypothermia is being considered. A special low-reading thermometer is essential to measure core or deep body temperature. Rectal temperature may be used or, for community studies, the temperature of freshly passed urine has been used. Hypothermia is a serious condition and carries a significant mortality. Various studies of elderly patients report mortalities of between 30 and 75%.

Causes (Table 8.4)

For hypothermia to develop, exposure to cold must occur but also thermoregulation must be impaired so that body temperature cannot be maintained. Subjects of any age may become hypothermic when exposed to extreme cold. However, several cross-sectional and longitudinal studies in the UK have shown an age-related decline in thermoregulation (and other aspects of autonomic function) in a high proportion of otherwise fit, elderly people. Any serious illness in an older person may also be associated with failure to maintain normal body temperature. Immobility and disease, especially the reduced body metabolism of myxoedema, increases the risk of hypothermia considerably, as does the administration of drugs such as chlorpromazine, barbiturates and benzodiazepines, which directly impair thermoregulation. In some countries, alcoholism is commonly associated with hypothermia.

Table 8.4 *Causes of hypothermia*

Exogenous	—cold exposure
	—poor housing, inadequate heating or clothing
Endogenous	—impaired temperature homeostasis
	—immobility
	—any serious illness in an elderly person especially hypothyroidism
	—drugs

Clinical features

Hypothermic subjects have a pale and waxy appearance. A puffy face, slow cerebration and a husky voice are often mistaken for myxoedema, but this appearance is totally reversible when the patients are rewarmed. The skin feels cold and shivering is often absent. Patients may appear apathetic and disorientated; they may have hallucinations or show paranoid features. Consciousness may be impaired if the core temperature is less than 32°C. In the presence of impaired consciousness, breathing is slow and shallow and may show features of Cheyne–Stokes respiration. The pulse is slow, indicating sinus bradycardia or slow atrial fibrillation. There is generalized muscle rigidity and diminished tendon reflexes. Many patients show an involuntary flapping tremor of their arms and legs. The common complications of hypothermia, pancreatitis and bronchopneumonia, often occur without any of the usual clinical signs.

Investigations show haemoconcentration, although the serum sodium is usually below the normal range. The serum potassium may be high or low, but may fall on rewarming, which increases the risks of cardiac dysrhythmias. Blood glucose levels are often high, because insulin is inactive in the cold, but fall on rewarming. The ECG commonly shows some degree of heart block and the characteristic 'J' wave, a deflection at the junction of the QRS and ST segments. Other cardiac dysrhythmias may also be seen with continuous ECG monitoring. The serum creatine kinase is often raised as a result of muscle damage while the serum amylase is often elevated and pancreatitis frequently found at post mortem examination.

Treatment

Treatment of mild hypothermia (32–35°C) is by slow rewarming in warm surroundings (e.g. 27°C). Patients should be well covered with blankets, with the aim of raising core temperature by 0.5°C per hour. Rapid rewarming is hazardous, causing extensive cutaneous vasodilatation, a fall in blood pressure and impaired tissue perfusion. Treatment of patients with severe hypothermia (less than 32°C) is best undertaken in intensive care surroundings whenever possible.

Attention to the patient's airway is essential and 28% oxygen is given to counteract arterial hypoxia. All patients should have their pulse, blood pressure and core temperature taken at frequent intervals, also their fluid balance measured and conscious level recorded. Cardiac monitoring will demonstrate the presence of dysrhythmias, which may need treatment. Warmed, intravenous fluids should be given cautiously; the central venous pressure may need to be measured to avoid overhydration. Gastric dilatation may be sufficiently pronounced to require nasogastric intubation, thereby preventing possible aspiration. Serum potassium may fall during rewarming, hence potassium supplements are often necessary to prevent additional cardiac dysrhythmias.

Intravenous broad-spectrum antibiotics should be given routinely to treat or prevent pneumonia, regardless of clinical signs. Intravenous hydrocortisone may also be given over the first 48 hours, though the precise benefits are not well established.

Prevention

Any patients who have suffered accidental hypothermia are at particular risk of its recurrence and therefore this vulnerable group should be carefully monitored in the future. Drugs with hypothermic actions should be used with caution and for as short a time as possible. Standards of housing should be improved wherever possible to ensure that the buildings are warm and free from draughts. Elderly people should be encouraged to heat their bedrooms in the winter and keep their windows closed. It may be necessary to request financial assistance from Social Services Departments for extra clothing, bedding or food.

NORMAL PRESSURE HYDROCEPHALUS

This uncommon condition is associated with fluctuating but progressive dementia, a spastic ataxic gait and incontinence of urine and faeces. As the name implies, hydrocephalus is present, usually of idiopathic origin, while the pressure within the cerebrospinal fluid (CSF) is normal. On CT scanning, prominent ventricular dilatation is seen without cortical atrophy. Treatment in the form of a shunt of the CSF away from the lateral ventricles sometimes brings dramatic benefit. Such surgery carries an appreciable morbidity. The pathophysiology of the condition and its response to treatment are poorly understood.

CHRONIC SUBDURAL HAEMATOMA

A chronic subdural haematoma occurs if one or more veins crossing the subdural space to reach the dural sinuses are torn. The collection of blood becomes encased by a highly vascular membrane and slowly enlarges as fluid moves into it across the osmotic gradient. Because some degree of cortical atrophy occurs with increasing age, the haematoma may become quite large before it causes neurological signs and symptoms.

It is caused by head injury, a common occurrence in elderly people, with their propensity to falls. The trauma may be quite trivial, especially if there is a disorder of haemostasis as well, or if a patient is taking anticoagulant therapy. A history of head injury may be missing in the presence of mental confusion or alcoholism, or in the absence of reliable witnesses. Symptoms may include confusion and impaired memory, mimicking dementia, sometimes with marked fluctuation of mental function and focal fits. In the later stages, the level of consciousness may fluctuate and lateralizing neurlogical signs, e.g. hemiparesis, may develop.

A high index of suspicion is needed to make this diagnosis which, unfortunately, is frequently missed during life. A plain skull radiograph may show displacement of a calcified pineal gland, which suggests the presence of a space-occupying lesion. However, CT scanning of the brain is the most effective method of diagnosis. Treatment by evacuation of the haematoma through a burr hole in the cranium is well tolerated and often produces dramatic improvement in neurological function.

CERVICAL SPONDYLOSIS

Cervical spondylosis describes degenerative changes in the cervical intervertebral discs, and secondary changes in adjacent vertebrae. As the intervertebral discs degenerate and lose volume, the intervertebral spaces become narrowed and the vertebral arteries, running cranially in the transverse foramina of the upper six cervical vertebrae, become kinked and tortuous. Osteophytes, which form as bony bars or spurs at the margins of the vertebral bodies, may project into the intervertebral foramina to compress the spinal nerve roots. Symptoms arising from cervical spondylosis may take the form of cervical root compression, cord compression or vertebrobasilar insufficiency.

Drop attacks may be precipitated by turning or extending the neck, and cause the patient to fall to the ground, with momentary or no loss of consciousness. Full recovery occurs immediately afterwards. They are thought to be due to vertebral artery compression leading to the momentary failure of an adequate blood supply to the reticular formation of the brain stem. The elderly cerebral circulation is particularly at risk in the presence of cervical spondylosis because of cerebral atherosclerosis and the age-related impairment of autoregulation of the cerebral circulation.

EPILEPSY

Epilepsy, presenting as 'black-outs' or recurrent falls, may occur in elderly patients as a result of cerebrovascular disease, as an effect of a cerebral tumour or of dementia. Patients usually lose consciousness; they may have convulsions and are often incontinent of urine. The history from an independent observer is most important in the diagnosis of this condition, which is usually readily controlled by anticonvulsant medication.

Chapter

9

Special Senses—Visual Loss and Deafness

VISUAL LOSS • CAUSES OF GRADUAL LOSS OF VISION • CAUSES OF SUDDEN LOSS OF VISION • DEAFNESS • COMMON AUDITORY PROBLEMS

Failing vision and impaired hearing are frequent accompaniments of later life. Steps must always be taken to minimize these defects as they may induce considerable sensory deprivation, which itself may cause much social isolation and contribute to mental confusion.

VISUAL LOSS

In the UK, it has been estimated that there are 300 000 people who are severely visually handicapped, 75% of them being of pensionable age. Visual loss may develop slowly and insidiously over a period of several months or occur suddenly (Table 9.1). Depending upon the cause, some restoration of vision may be achieved by treatment. In the UK, blindness is caused chiefly by three diseases: macular degeneration, glaucoma and cataract.

Age-related changes in vision that can be measured include: (i) reduced powers of accommodation (presbyopia); and (ii) a reduction in visual acuity. Accommodation is the ability of the lens to become 'fatter' and focus near objects on the surface of the retina. Powers of accommodation are progressively reduced throughout adult life, due to many factors including a reduction in the elasticity of the lens substance and the progressive growth of the lens itself. Visual acuity remains

Table 9.1 *Causes of visual loss*

Gradual	*Sudden*
Senile macular degeneration Cataract Glaucoma—open angle	Arterial occlusion Venous occlusion Glaucoma—closed angle Retinal detachment Diabetic retinopathy Cerebrovascular disease

fairly constant until the fifth decade of life after which a gradual reduction is observed.

Physical examination of the eyes must always include inspection of any spectacles used. Elderly people often have difficulty in going to opticians and their spectacles may have been bought years before and are therefore unlikely to correct current refractive difficulties. On a simpler level, they may be broken, dirty or even lost! Examination of the external eye may reveal corneal opacities, iritis, pupillary changes or the evidence of past eye surgery. The ophthalmoscope is used to visualize any lens opacities that may be present, as well as the optic disc and retinal vessels. Distance acuity is tested with a Snellen chart at 6 metres, while standard reading test type cards are useful for near acuity. Visual field testing by confrontation is essential for determining visual field defects.

Blindness

The current statutory definition of blindness is 'that a person should be so blind as to be unable to perform any work for which eye sight is essential'. In general, a person is eligible for registration if the visual acuity is 3/60 or less in both eyes. If the visual fields are impaired, visual acuity may be better, though the patient is still registerable as blind. To be registered as partially sighted, the patient must have a vision of 6/60 or worse in both eyes, although again, visual acuity may be better if the visual fields are appreciably restricted.

The registration of a patient as being blind or partially sighted needs to be authorized by a consultant ophthalmologist and this confers various benefits and entitlements to the patient (most of which are not applicable or appropriate to elderly patients who lose their sight in later life). In 1986, 185 000 people were registered blind and 81 000 as partially sighted. It has been estimated that 60% of those who are registered blind have at least one additional handicap, e.g. diabetes, physical disability or deafness.

Consequences of blindness

Blindness may be catastrophic if it occurs in later life. Visual loss may totally obliterate a patient's self-confidence and usually prevents independence. Mobility is often restricted and social isolation may result. If such a person lives alone, complete self-care is rarely possible without additional social support. An elderly person who has become blind is seldom able to become familiar with Braille. Reading is therefore restricted to large print books, using low vision aids, or listening to recorded tapes of people reading books or newspapers out loud ('talking books').

CAUSES OF GRADUAL LOSS OF VISION

Senile macular degeneration

The macula, concerned with central vision, may be subject to degenerative changes which cause an insidious loss of vision due to bilateral central scotomata. It may appear swollen with exudate or covered by blood or haemorrhagic residues, often with pigmentation present. These changes are thought to occur as a result of tearing between the membrane layers and the retina, with consequent new vessel formation. The condition is probably inherited and may occasionally occur in young adults. No treatment is able to halt or reverse these changes at present. Patients may be helped initially by using strong reading glasses or a magnifying glass for close work.

Cataract

The lens is an avascular and transparent structure and its cells, (excluding those of the anterior epithelium) which lose their nuclei early in development, are therefore subsequently unable to divide. Any abnormality in its structure or metabolism causes the lens to become opaque. Local irregularities in the lens structure are visualized with an ophthalmoscope either in the centre of the lens, where they form a silhouette against the red fundus reflex, or on the periphery, where they are seen as flakes, dots or sector-shaped opacities. Some degree of lens opacity is found in the majority of people over 60 years old and cataract formation is thought to be a genetically determined exaggeration of the normal ageing process. Subjects particularly prone to the development of cataracts are those with diabetes, gout or on long-term steroid therapy. Cataracts may be bilateral, but there are often marked differences between the two sides.

If interference with vision by central opacities occurs, temporary improvement may be achieved by providing spectacles for increasing myopia, or by dilating the pupils. As opacification of the lens is irreversible, the only treatment possible is its removal by surgery. Surgery can be performed at any age and at any stage in cataract development. However, it is generally advised when the cataract produces poor vision sufficient to interfere with normal daily activities. Modern surgical practice is to implant an acrylic lens at the time of surgery, which eliminates the optical distortion caused by the thick post-cataract spectacles that previously were necessary.

Glaucoma—open angle

Glaucoma affects 1 in 200 people over 40 years of age and is a common cause of new blind registration. Seventy-five per cent of all patients with primary glaucoma have open angle glaucoma, responsible for an insidious loss of vision which may not be noticed until late in the course of the disease.

The normal eye maintains an intra-ocular pressure (IOP) of approximately 15 mmHg, which represents the difference between the rate of fluid (aqueous) secretion into the eye and the bulk flow of aqueous out of the eye. Eyes with IOPs greater than 21 mmHg (two standard deviations above the mean) are considered to have elevated intra-ocular pressure. Open angle glaucoma is thought to be the result of a progressive increase in the resistance of the aqueous to leave the eye, via the outflow system, which is situated in the angle of the anterior chamber. Prolonged elevation of IOP, detected by tonometry, produces compression of the head of the optic nerve and hence defects in the visual field. An arcuate scotoma is produced initially, extending from the blind spot to the periphery in the nasal field, and only in the latter stages does this involve the central field vision. Examination of the eye reveals an ischaemic white optic disc, which is 'cupped' in appearance.

Treatment should be directed by an ophthalmologist and depends on the extent of visual loss. Its aim is to reduce IOP to within the normal range. Eye drops (e.g. pilocarpine, adrenaline and guanethidine) act to reduce outflow resistance, but occasionally surgery is required, where a permanent fistula is created in the iris between the anterior chamber and the subconjunctival space, allowing easier egress of the aqueous from the eye.

CAUSES OF SUDDEN LOSS OF VISION

Arterial occlusion

Occlusion of the central retinal artery by thrombus formation or emboli from the carotid vessels or from the heart causes sudden and complete loss of vision in that eye. Fundoscopy shows the retinal arteries as narrow threads, while the whole fundus appears milky white as the oedematous retina loses its transparency. After a day or two, a 'cherry red spot' appears at the macula, where the retina is at its thinnest and the red choroid shows through. When only a branch of the central artery is occluded, only the corresponding sector of retina is affected, leaving an appropriate scotoma.

Occlusion of the central retinal artery is a common sequel to giant-cell arteritis, which involves the aterioles round the optic disc. A raised erythrocyte sedimentation rate will confirm this diagnosis. Treatment with systemic steroids will reduce the oedema of the optic disc but, of greater importance, prevent a similar occurrence in the other eye.

Venous occlusion

The central retinal vein may be occluded by pressure of its escorting artery at the optic disc, especially in the presence of venous congestion. Hypertensive and arteriosclerotic patients are at particular risk of this. Though loss of sight is a little less abrupt and less complete than with arterial occlusion, fundoscopy shows a mass of irregular haemorrhages scattered throughout the retina, the veins themselves appearing tortuous and engorged. New vessels are formed on the iris as a result of retinal hypoxia and acute secondary glaucoma may therefore develop to obliterate any vision remaining.

Closed angle glaucoma

The sudden development of raised IOP not only causes blurring of vision but also severe pain in the eye, often accompanied by nausea and occasionally vomiting. Such acute glaucoma presents with an irregularly dilated pupil, which is non-reactive to light, and a cloudy oedematous cornea while the surrounding conjuctiva is reddened. It is caused by the iris making contact with the back of the cornea and obliterating the peripheral recess of the anterior chamber, thereby preventing the aqueous from escaping into the outflow system.

Since an attack of acute glaucoma may be precipitated by pupil dilatation, emergency treatment in the form of pilocarpine drops, instilled into the eye every few minutes, may help by constricting the pupil. In addition to potent analgesia, acetazolamide, a carbonic anhydrase inhibitor, given intramuscularly, will assist by inhibiting aqueous production.

Surgery may be required for emergency decompression, but is always recommended as future prophylaxis after an acute episode has settled. A small hole is made in the iris root to allow free passage of aqueous between anterior and posterior chambers. As closed angle glaucoma is likely to affect both eyes, it is accepted practice that peripheral iridectomies are performed prophylactically on both eyes.

Retinal detachment

Rupture of the pigment epithelium allows the vitreous to seep between it and the underlying rods and cones and to separate the two layers, so that the visual layer is displaced forwards as a retinal detachment. Such ruptures generally occur in degenerate patches at the retinal periphery and may occur spontaneously in the ageing eye. Retinal detachment has been described as a curtain descending (or ascending, if the detachment started above), central vision being lost completely when the detachment spreads across the macula area. Treatment is by skilled early surgery, sealing the retina back to the choroid all round the original tear.

Diabetic retinopathy

Diabetic retinopathy is characterized by the presence of haemorrhages, exudates and micro-aneurysms. In elderly patients, it is often complicated by the coincident signs of retinal arteriosclerosis. The diabetic changes may be arrested by laser treatment, but visual loss will occur if the macula region is involved or if massive haemorrhage into the vitreous occurs.

Cerebrovascular disease

Vision may be affected at several sites in a patient who has had a stroke. Cerebral thrombosis involving the occipital cortex will produce cortical blindness of the contralateral homonymous field. Optic tract lesions will similarly produce contralateral visual field defects, varying with the amount of damage, but maximal with a homonymous hemianopia. Transient retinal artery occlusions producing temporary blindness are sometimes associated with contralateral hemiparesis, due to recurrent emboli from atheromatous plaques in the common carotid arteries.

DEAFNESS

Deafness is defined as the loss of hearing, regardless of its severity. It is one of the commonest disabilities, the incidence rising dramatically with increasing age. Many population surveys have estimated the prevalence of deafness to be up to a third of the population over 65 years of age, with at least 50% of subjects not having sought medical advice about their hearing loss. Impaired hearing impairs the ability to communicate and is a significant disability. Being unable to communicate with others often leads to loss of independence and social isolation, and may be associated with the development of psychological disorders, such as depression, anxiety and paranoid tendencies. Deafness is still perceived negatively as a disability; sufferers often feel stigmatized by their disability, which is poorly appreciated and may gain little sympathy from others.

Age-related changes in the auditory system

Physiological effects of ageing need to be distinguished from superimposed pathological changes of age-associated disease. There are several functional abnormalities associated with the ageing auditory system:

1. An impaired sensitivity to high frequency sounds (presbyacusis).
2. Development of tinnitus (both are discussed further below).
3. Perception of loudness is progressively impaired.
4. Detection of direction of sound and its localization are also impaired.
5. A decline in sound discrimination, especially of speech.

These physiological effects may be a result of degenerative changes affecting the inner ear, as well as due to cortical changes, where the rate of information processing from afferent stimuli is reduced.

Deafness is often multifactorial but is traditionally classified as *conductive*, where there is an impediment to the conduction of sound waves through the external to the middle ear and *sensorineural*, where the defect is central to the oval window.

Management of deafness

Before assessing the nature of a patient's deafness, it is essential to inspect the ears and exclude the presence of wax in the external auditory canals. If present, its removal may produce a dramatic improvement in communication. It is helpful when talking with any deaf person, especially if elderly, to have a face-to-face conversation in surroundings where auditory and visual distractions are minimal, and to speak clearly and more slowly than normal. This is particularly important for people who have become deaf in later life, who generally will not have developed the skills of sign language or lip reading. Gestures may also be used as a supplement to speech, to aid communication.

If a hearing aid is available, the elderly person should be encouraged to wear it (after checking it is in working order, e.g. the batteries are not flat and the plastic tubing intact and not blocked by wax). A portable speech amplifier (or even an ear trumpet!) is helpful if a deaf person does not have one available. These sound magnifiers, however, have a major disadvantage and one that is responsible for many people not using them in their daily lives. They magnify *all* sound non-specifically, so that not only speech but also much extraneous noise is similarly magnified, the result often being most unpleasant for the recipient.

In the home, a flashing light may be installed as a substitute for the doorbell and for other alarm systems, if a deaf person lives alone. Various adaptors may be installed to magnify telephone conversations and to bring sound from the television or radio direct to the ear of the listener.

COMMON AUDITORY PROBLEMS

Presbyacusis

Presbyacusis is the age-related loss of pure tone hearing in the higher frequencies. It is often accompanied by abnormal loudness perception, so that, although an elderly person may be hard of hearing, noisy surroundings are poorly tolerated. There is considerable variation in the degree of high-frequency loss. Aetiological mechanisms remain speculative.

Tinnitus

Tinnitus is a common problem, increasing in incidence with increasing age; it has been estimated that at least 10% of men and women over 65 years old experience it. Tinnitus is thought to be an 'internal noise' generated within the auditory system and is not necessarily associated with hearing loss. It causes distress in proportion to its intensity but may be modified by a patient's mental or physical health. Many drugs have been implicated in causing auditory damage with associated tinnitus, but none are helpful in its treatment. For patients who are also deaf, a hearing aid may relieve both problems, whereas if hearing is not sufficiently impaired, a hearing-aid type of instrument, called a 'tinnitus masker', may be used. This instrument which generates constant sound and masks the tinnitus, even when it is removed may suppress the tinnitus for a short time afterwards. The patient adjusts the volume of the masker and wears it like a hearing aid, for long periods.

Otosclerosis

Otosclerosis is an inherited condition and should be suspected in those whose deafness is more severe than would be expected from age alone. Deafness is bilateral and bone conduction of sound is more effective than conduction through air. It is caused by the foot plate of the stapes bone becoming adherent to the oval window, thus interfering with the transmission of sound through to the inner ear. Specialist ENT advice should be sought for consideration of stapedectomy.

Dizziness

Dizziness is a very frequent complaint of elderly patients but one which often eludes an accurate diagnosis. It may be associated with cardiovascular insufficiency, as occurs in postural hypotension (*see* p. 100), or the presence of cardiac dysrhythmias or even severe anaemia. However, dizziness may be experienced together with vertigo, the illusion of movement, when it may be caused by a defect within the ear or central connecting pathways. Transient cerebral ischaemic episodes and vertebrobasilar insufficiency are also commonly implicated. Menière's disease is associated with episodes of a sudden onset of severe dizziness, accompanied by nausea and sometimes vomiting; it may also present as unilateral progressive deafness.

Drugs and dizziness

Although the ototoxicity of aminoglycosides is well known, other drugs are often implicated in the aetiology of dizziness. They may increase the risk of postural hypotension and/or the incidence of cardiac dysrhythmias (e.g. digoxin, diuretics, β-blockers, antidepressants and phenothiazines). Frail postural and balance mechanisms may be further destabilized by sedation from benzodiazepines and other hypnotics, or even by alcohol.

Chapter 10

Falls and Immobility

POSTURE • CAUSES OF FALLS • CONSEQUENCES OF FALLS • IMMOBILITY FACTORS

People of any age may trip over an uneven floor surface, especially if vision is impaired by poor lighting. However, older people are more at risk of falling than younger adults. The maintenance of an erect posture is less efficient with increasing age (*see* below). Elderly people are less able to correct unwanted body movement; cardiovascular and neurological deficits may further exacerbate failing homeostatic mechanisms. Mechanical problems involving the muscles and joints of the legs may conspire to make postural stability even more precarious.

POSTURE

Sway and control of posture

The maintenance of a stable erect posture is complex, requiring that the body, with its high centre of gravity, is balanced over a small area of and between the feet. The cerebellum and brain stem coordinate this activity via sensory signals from the skin, muscles and joints. Visual stimuli and sensation arising from the vestibular apparatus also contribute. The effector part of this activity comprises the anti-gravity muscles, limb and spinal joints and their neurological control. To stand completely still requires a recognition of minor degrees of change in position and their immediate correction by the anti-gravity muscles.

Postural sway, observed as body movement while subjects attempt to stand quite still, is a normal reflex phenomenon, delegated to the realms of the unconscious throughout most of life. It is poor in early childhood, reaches a maximum in early adulthood, but progressively deteriorates from the 50s onwards (Fig. 10.1). Increased postural sway

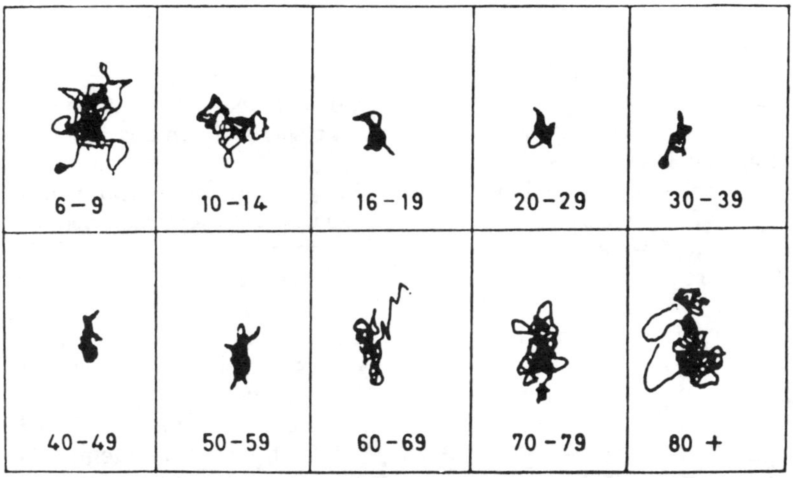

6–9 | 10–14 | 16–19 | 20–29 | 30–39

40–49 | 50–59 | 60–69 | 70–79 | 80 +

Figure 10.1 Typical tracings of body sway from each age group in the direct vision/stance test (*after* Sheldon, 1963)

may be due to mismatching of sensory information associated with ageing or disease affecting vestibular, proprioceptive and visual information, together with impaired righting reflexes. This phenomenon forms the basis of the Romberg test. Falls are common in elderly people, but they are generally caused by additional paroxysmal events which aggravate an already impaired system of postural control. Increased sway, demonstrating impaired postural control, is most evident in elderly people with a history of falls, whether due to giddiness, loss of balance or drop attacks.

CAUSES OF FALLS

People may fall for various reasons and a careful history and examination is essential to determine the cause of each fall (Table 10.1). Often, a combination of factors is responsible, some of which are reversible by treatment, such patients being rendered less likely to fall in the future by treatment.

Table 10.1 *Causes of falls*

Environmental	e.g. Slip mats, uneven paving, objects on floor, poor lighting
Intrinsic	
—defective sensory input	Poor vision, peripheral neuropathy, vestibular disorders
—defective neurological control	Epilepsy, cerebellar ataxia, stroke, Parkinsonism, 'drop attacks'
—defective cardiovascular control	Cardiac dysrhythmias—sudden bradycardia or tachycardia, complete heart block
	Hypotension—after myocardial infarct, pulmonary embolus, or massive haemorrhage —postural hypotension
	Effort syncope—severe aortic stenosis, micturition/defaecation syncope
	Carotid sinus hypersensitivity
—musculoskeletal disorders	Myopathies, e.g. osteomalacia
	Unstable joints, e.g. osteoarthritis, rheumatoid arthritis
Drug therapy	e.g. Drugs causing postural hypotension, hypokalaemia, excessive sedation, Parkinsonism

External causes

As remarked above, trips on uneven flooring may happen to anyone. Equally, objects on the floor or pets may be unnoticed or unseen because of inadequate lighting. However, such reasons may be offered by a patient as a means of justifying a fall that is not otherwise explicable. Much tact is therefore needed to distinguish between what actually happened from what 'probably' happened.

Intrinsic causes 1. Defective sensory input

Visual defects such as lens opacities, retinal degeneration or visual field defects may increase the likelihood of obstacles being overlooked. If dizziness, i.e. a false sensation of movement, precedes the fall, it may suggest vestibular dysfunction (*see* Chapter 9). (True vertigo is, however, rare.) Loss of tactile sensation or joint-position sense in the feet may cause problems in walking and may be associated with a high stepping or broad-based gait. Such deficits may equally increase the risk of falling.

2. Defective neurological control

The history of an epileptic fit is sufficient to explain a fall where a witness is on hand. If direct observations are not available, such a diagnosis must be made with care. Epilepsy occurring in later life is usually due to cerebrovascular disease, although a cerebral tumour should always be excluded. Similarly, the development of muscle weakness after a stroke or a TIA may be sufficient to cause a fall. The presence of cerebellar ataxia or Parkinsonism is associated with characteristic gaits and postural instability. Drop attacks occur, as their name implies, suddenly and without warning, with momentary or no loss of consciousness. There is no neurological deficit afterwards. Drop attacks may be precipitated by neck movements, interrupting the blood supply to the brain (*see* Chapter 8).

3. Defective cardiovascular control

Intermittent cardiac dysrhythmias causing falls may produce subjective palpitations beforehand. These may be demonstrated by continuous ambulatory ECG monitoring. Many short episodes may be symptom-free, but those which are associated with temporary but significant reductions in cardiac output may cause dizziness or a black-out. Drug treatment of cardiac dysrhythmias is the same as for younger patients, with attention to any dose reductions needed, because of altered drug handling in the elderly (*see* Chapter 4). The indications for cardiac pacing are the same as for younger patients.

Any conditions where hypotension or a reduced cardiac output are produced will cause syncope and falls. Myocardial infarction (often with an atypical presentation), pulmonary embolism or massive haemorrhage may all have other features in the history or examination suggestive of these conditions, with falls being a consequence of them.

Postural hypotension (orthostatic hypotension)

Postural hypotension is common in elderly people and may be defined as a fall in systolic pressure of 20 mmHg or more on assuming an erect stance. It often causes unsteadiness, dizziness and faintness, especially after rising from bed in the morning (or during the night). However, some patients with postural hypotension may be asymptomatic, because autoregulatory mechanisms preserve a normal cerebral blood flow. The blood pressure should be recorded when the patient has lain down for about five minutes or more, and then after standing for two minutes. If the systolic pressure is less than 80–90 mmHg, syncope will often result.

The regulation of blood pressure depends on reflex mechanisms involving cardiac output and peripheral resistance. Heart rate, which influences cardiac output, is controlled by baroreceptor reflexes originating from the carotid sinus; a fall in blood pressure leads to a rise in heart rate. Peripheral resistance is dependent on vasoconstrictor tone mediated by the sympathetic nervous system. Normally on standing after lying supine, blood is initially pooled in the abdomen and legs, with a reduction in the return of blood to the right side of the heart. However, systemic arterial pressure is maintained by an almost simultaneous decrease in parasympathetic activity (leading to cardiac acceleration) and an increase in sympathetic activity (causing vasoconstriction of arteries and veins).

If these mechanisms are less effective, as occurs with increasing age, or they are combined with conditions that reduce the preload to the heart (e.g. hypovolaemia or reduced venous return) or cause arterial vasodilatation (reducing after-load to the heart), the systemic blood pressure will fall on assuming an erect stance (Table 10.2). Drug therapy is frequently implicated in the development of symptomatic postural hypotension, overcoming the limited reserves of an ageing homeostatic system (see Table 10.3). Drugs which act either on the baroreceptor reflex or directly on the blood vessels, unless essential, should be discontinued whenever possible.

Table 10.2 *Causes of postural hypotension*

Impaired baroreceptor reflexes	Ageing Disease of central nervous system* Polyneuropathies Prolonged bed rest
Hypovolaemia	Dehydration Haematemesis Addison's disease
Reduced venous return	Impaired mobility Varicose veins Micturition/defaecation syncope
Vasodilatation	
Drug therapy	

* e.g. Parkinsonism, diabetes, tabes dorsalis, cerebellar degeneration

Table 10.3 *Drugs which may cause postural hypotension*

Hypotensive agents (esp. diuretics, β-blockers and vasodilators)
Tranquillizers (esp. phenothiazines, benzodiazepines and butyrophenones)
Tricyclic antidepressants
L-dopa
Alcohol

Management of postural hypotension depends on identifying which combination of factors are responsible for it. As well as stopping or reducing any drugs that could be implicated, any underlying pathology should be treated and fluid depletion corrected. Slow and gradual changes in posture should be encouraged to allow time for reflex adjustments to occur. Prolonged bed rest should be avoided and physical activity encouraged. Pooling of blood on assuming the upright position may be prevented by mechanical means through the use of full-length elastic stockings. Elevation of the head of the patient's bed allows reactive vasoconstriction in the peripheral vessels, as well as sodium retention, which is lost during recumbency.

Specific drug therapy is limited but the mineralocorticoid, fludrocortisone, by increasing sodium retention and expanding the blood volume, may be used with some improvement in symptoms. However, it produces potassium loss, so serum electrolytes need to be monitored regularly and potassium supplements given when necessary.

Effort syncope

Exertion in the presence of severe aortic stenosis may produce a fall in cardiac output, and hence a fall in cerebral perfusion, sufficient to cause syncope at any age. Systolic cardiac murmurs are common in elderly patients; therefore, in patients who have had falls, great care should be taken before making this diagnosis, which should only be made after confirmation by cardiac investigations, e.g. echocardiography.

Syncope has been reported after coughing or straining during micturition and defaecation. It is thought to arise because of failure of venous return to the heart from raised intrathoracic or intra-abdominal pressure. Circulatory changes similar to those accompanying a Valsalva manoeuvre have been demonstrated. Elderly men with prostatism and nocturia may frequently fall at night. The effects of straining to pass urine, postural hypotension and the administration of hypnotics may combine to cause such falls.

Carotid sinus hypersensitivity

Pressure on the carotid sinus may lead to syncope at any age. Carotid sinus hypersensitivity can give rise to extreme sinus bradycardia or even asystole and may be precipitated by drugs, including digoxin and propranolol. It is a rare cause of falls. It may be reproduced by carotid sinus compression with continuous ECG monitoring. However, this should only be done when necessary and with great care.

4. Musculoskeletal disorders

Any weakness of locomotor function may produce sufficient postural instability to increase the risk of falling. The combination of degenerative joint disease and surrounding weak musculature and ligaments may be responsible for frequent episodes where the joints 'just give way'. Such times occur typically while rising from a chair or climbing stairs. Muscle weakness alone may also be responsible for falls. Myopathies due to disturbances of potassium homeostasis (hyper- and hypokalaemia), thyrotoxicosis and alcoholism are occasionally seen. Osteomalacia is associated with weakness of the proximal muscles, causing difficulty walking and the characteristic waddling gait (*see* p. 132). Such a myopathy and other symptoms can be readily corrected by administration of vitamin D.

Iatrogenic causes (drug therapy)

Finally, iatrogenic causes for falls must always be excluded. Discontinuing a drug that may be responsible for causing significant postural hypotension and falls related to standing is often a very simple but rewarding exercise (*see* Table 10.3). Hypokalaemia caused by diuretics or laxative abuse may, by causing muscle weakness, be responsible for frequent falls and impaired mobility. Equally, drugs causing excessive sedation or extra-pyramidal side-effects may also contribute to the development of instability and falls, by reducing neurological surveillence or the resultant muscle efficiency in postural control.

At present, the changes of an ageing nervous system cannot be reversed. However, it is often the addition of other problems, e.g. cardiac dysrhythmias or hypovolaemia due to diuretics, which may be eminently treatable, but serve as 'the last straw' to compromise the postural stability of an elderly person.

CONSEQUENCES OF FALLS

The important sequelae of falls are summarized in Table 10.4. The major complication of frequent falls is a loss of confidence in an elderly person's ability to be independent. Such patients may take to their beds and become completely immobile. Alternatively, if they have fallen out of doors, fear of further falls may render them housebound.

Table 10.4 *Possible sequelae of falls*

Loss of confidence and immobility
Soft tissue injuries
Fractures
Subdural haematoma
Hypothermia
Dehydration
Pressure sores
Bronchopneumonia
Burns

The fall itself may be associated with bruising, which can be extensive or trivial. However, the discomfort and stiffness it produces can, if untreated, severely limit mobility, causing further problems. The possibility that an injury to the head has occurred at the time of the fall should raise the suspicion of a subdural haematoma (*see* p. 84). Fractures of the hip, wrist or ribs may also occur as a direct result of a fall and need specific treatment. Falling near an open fire or close to a radiator and being subsequently unable to move can result in extensive burns. Scalding with hot water can similarly cause much damage to the skin. Burns have a high mortality in the elderly, even with expert care.

If a person has fallen and, living alone, is unable to get up again, she may lie on a cold, hard floor for many hours before assistance is at hand. During this time, such patients are at great risk of developing hypothermia, dehydration, pressure sores, rhabdomyolysis (leading to renal failure) and bronchopneumonia. Hence the mortality of falls in the elderly is considerable and steps must be taken wherever possible to make falling less likely.

Physiotherapy and the provision of walking aids may help many patients who have fallen recover confidence and a safer walking pattern. It is always as well to be sure that such patients can manage to get up from the floor, if they are unfortunate enough to have subsequent falls. If this is not feasible, the occupational therapist may advise them about a portable alarm or an alarm-call system, which can be installed at home.

IMMOBILITY FACTORS

As elderly people grow older, many become less able to move around independently such that, as time goes by, they go outdoors less and less. A common presentation of a sick elderly person is the complaint that she has 'gone off her legs', becoming bed-fast or chair-fast. In such a situation, she is unable to lead an independent life, which places increased demands on those around her or on the Social Services Departments. It is important to discover from the history just what activities are no longer possible, that were previously manageable (and, if possible, what else happened at the same time, to account for this). Possible causes are legion (Table 10.5) and while only some may be completely reversible, most can be improved considerably with specific treatment.

Table 10.5 *Causes of immobility*

Local pain from—bones	Osteoporosis, Paget's, bony metastases, fractures, osteomalacia
—joints	Osteoarthritis, rheumatoid arthritis
—muscles and soft tissues	Polymyalgia rheumatica, painful feet, peripheral vascular disease
—neurological	Stroke, Parkinsonism, peripheral neuropathy, cerebellar ataxia
Systemic—cardiovascular	Reduced exercise tolerance, postural hypotension
—endocrine	Myxoedema, thyrotoxicosis, diabetes, osteomalacia, Cushing's syndrome
—metabolic	Hypokalaemia
Psychological	Fear of falling, depression, dementia
Drug therapy	

NB Causes of temporary immobility may become permanent, if untreated

Any temporary decline in mobility may, unless adequately treated, become self-perpetuating. For instance, a fall, for whatever reason, may be associated with bruising and stiffness. It is not unreasonable for a person to rest in bed afterwards, but such immobility may cause the pain and stiffness to worsen, with the possibility of bronchopneumonia, pressure sores and incontinence developing subsequently. Similarly, temporary inactivity and bed rest with a chest infection may, if continued too long, impair an elderly person's ability to regain their previous level of independence.

Causes of impaired mobility and their treatment

Local causes

Pain arising from bone, joints or soft tissues is a common cause of impaired mobility. Specific causes of bone pain are covered elsewhere and include osteoporosis, osteomalacia and Paget's disease (*see* Chapter 12), pain arising from bony metastases (*see* p. 155) and fractures. Similarly, pain from the arthropathies may increase in severity and cause mobility to decline (*see* Chapter 11).

Peripheral vascular disease and polymyalgia rheumatica may also limit mobility and, when severe, render a patient virtually immobile. Even trivial conditions (for younger patients) of painful bunions and corns may play a significant role in reducing mobility. The development of pressure sores on the heels during an acute illness may be sufficiently painful to hinder attempts at walking early in the recovery phase and prolong the period of dependency.

Many neurological problems may also be responsible for a decline in mobility, e.g. hemiplegic patients may be unable to roll over in bed unaided or, merely, be unable to climb stairs safely. Parkinsonism, cerebellar ataxia and peripheral neuropathy will also impair mobility and encourage the development of problems associated with permanent immobility (*see* above).

Systemic causes

Malaise and lethargy are vague symptoms of generalized weakness. Poor exercise tolerance of patients with cardiac failure or after a myocardial infarct will severely reduce mobility. The development of postural hypotension on standing up, from whatever cause, will equally act as a strong disincentive to move about! Severe anaemia, whether microcytic or macrocytic, will also reduce exercise tolerance and may precipitate cardiac failure. Uncontrolled diabetes mellitus, or over- or under-activity of the thyroid and adrenal glands, may present as lethargy and immobility and are all eminently treatable. Osteomalacia is often associated not only with bone pain but proximal muscle weakness; both problems are reversed with vitamin D supplements. Hypokalaemia is a potent reason for muscle weakness and may be caused by increased renal loss of potassium from renal disease or diuretic therapy. Loss of gastrointestinal fluid from vomiting and diarrhoea will also cause potassium loss and require specific replacement.

Psychological causes

Fear of repeated falling, which in some cases is understandable, may totally immobilize many elderly people. In such cases, understanding the reason for the falls and, wherever possible, removing their cause will lessen the associated fear and anxiety. A short course of rehabilitation may be needed to restore muscle strength and re-educate balance, thereby improving patients' confidence in their own abilities.

There will be some immobile patients for whom no particular cause will be found for their immobility. They may simply appear not to wish to move around and passively accept all help offered in their self-care. Patients who are demented may show such inertia in the later stages of their illness. However, other treatable forms of mental illness may present in a similar way. Patients who are depressed may be sufficiently withdrawn and retarded to be found to be unable to move about freely or care for themselves. It is important to recognize such patients, presenting with pseudodementia, as they can usually be returned to normal after their depression has been treated. Rarely, patients with organic brain disease, especially affecting the frontal lobes, may present with immobility and require treatment directed to the specific cause of the disease.

Drug therapy

Drugs are potent causes both of falls and impaired mobility in the elderly. This iatrogenic disease is regrettably common, accounting for 10–15% of all hospital admissions (*see* Chapter 4). Such drugs can often be discontinued without major problems developing, or alternate therapy introduced without the offending side-effects.

Chapter

11

Joint Disease and Medical Aspects of Orthopaedic Surgery

OSTEOARTHRITIS • RHEUMATOID ARTHRITIS • OTHER ARTHROPATHIES • MEDICAL ASPECTS OF HIP SURGERY IN ELDERLY PATIENTS • MEDICAL MANAGEMENT OF THE ELDERLY ORTHOPAEDIC PATIENT

Painful joints are the cause of much pain and ill health and form a major cause of immobility and falls in the elderly. Osteoarthritis and rheumatoid arthritis are common and will be considered in some detail. Medical aspects of orthopaedic surgery, especially where fractures are repaired or joints replaced, will also be discussed; they are of vital importance to maximize the benefits of this treatment option and improve the quality of life for those elderly people who need them.

OSTEOARTHRITIS

Degenerative joint disease is almost universal with advancing years. There is much debate about whether osteoarthritis is an exaggerated reflection of the ageing process or a separate disease entity. It is a condition characterized by loss of articular cartilage and remodelling of the underlying subchondral bone. X-ray surveys of the elderly population have shown evidence of osteoarthritis in over 80%, but less than a quarter of subjects have joint symptoms. Osteoarthritis is age-related though not caused by ageing, and is responsible for a large burden of suffering and disability in the community, especially among the elderly. Factors concerned with its incidence, apart from increasing age, are previous disease of and trauma to joints, obesity and metabolic factors, e.g. achronosis and hyperuricaemia. In such cases, the osteoarthritis may be classed as secondary.

Cartilage—as hyaline cartilage in the synovial joints and fibrocartilage in the intervertebral discs and spinal articulations—undergoes chemical and structural changes throughout the normal life span and is the subject of much research. Articular cartilage is bluish white and almost transparent in young subjects, but with increasing age, becomes yellowy brown in colour and progressively opaque. With advancing age, the articular surface becomes uneven and shows the presence of fibrillation. Clefts and fissures are formed and eburnation of underlying bone and cyst formation occur in the subchondral marrow spaces. The intervertebral discs of fibrocartilage also show age-related degeneration. The nucleus pulposus becomes more fibrous and acquires a granular age pigment, while the inner part of the annulus becomes frayed. Tears in the intervertebral discs occur at points of particular mechanical stress, especially in the posterior part of the annulus fibrosus of L4 and L5 discs.

Degenerative disease of the spine occurs with similar degenerative changes to those of the peripheral joints but with additional degenerative changes in the intervertebral discs. Its incidence is higher in men than women and there is a clear relationship with heavy manual work. Other predisposing factors are postural disorders and kyphoscoliosis.

Clinical features

Osteoarthritis is strikingly variable in its patterns, presentations and outcome. Typical symptoms and signs include joint pain and crepitus, inactivity stiffness and joint deformity, often unaccompanied by signs of inflammation. Movement of the joint is restricted and pain is induced at the extremes of joint movement. Symptoms are often related to joint use and may fluctuate for no particular reason from very severe to painless at different times. All parts of the spine may be involved and the large synovial joints of the lower limbs (hips and knees) are more commonly affected than those of the upper limbs.

X-ray changes of osteoarthritis of synovial joints are joint space narrowing due to loss of cartilage, sclerosis of juxta-articular bone (eburnation) and the formation of osteophytes and bone cysts, caused by bone remodelling. Symptoms are very poorly correlated with radiographic appearances.

Histological examination of osteoarthritic joints shows evidence of low-grade chronic synovitis, characterized by patch infiltration of mononuclear cells in the synovium and thick clear effusions containing predominately mononuclear cells and fragments of cartilage. Whether such inflammation is the cause or result of the damaged cartilage found in osteoarthritic joints remains the subject of much debate and ongoing research.

Primary generalized osteoarthrosis

First described by Kellgren and Moore, primary generalized osteoarthritis may be distinguished from the various types of secondary osteoarthritis. It is a relatively benign condition affecting predominately women, initially at around the time of the menopause. It causes a symmetrical arthritis of the distal interphalangeal joints of the index and middle fingers (Heberden's nodes) and any of the proximal interphalangeal joints (Bouchard's nodes). Other joints may be affected including the apophyseal joints of the spine.

Treatment of osteoarthritis

There is no treatment known to have a beneficial effect on the changes seen in osteoarthritis. However, as the symptoms fluctuate and may settle spontaneously, management must be directed at palliating them and both maintaining and improving function of the joints to minimize permanent disability.

Patient education

Depression and anxiety are frequent accompaniments to the onset of pain from osteoarthritis (or any other pain). Both factors lower the threshold of pain and may therefore need to be addressed separately. Understanding the natural history of the condition may help to remove the fear of future incapacity. It is often helpful for patients to know that normal activities do not 'wear out' joints or cause progressive disease. Those who maintain their social and physical activities remain mobile and independent for longer. Obese patients with osteoarthritis of the hip and knee may suffer less pain if they reduce their weight and maintain their weight reduction.

Physical methods

To relieve joint pain, physical methods including local heat, ice packs, interferential (electrical) therapy and hydrotherapy, may be combined with active exercises to strengthen the surrounding muscles and increase the range of joint movement. Simple aids that alter the mechanical stress on damaged joints may also provide great relief. For example, a walking stick, used on the opposite side to an osteoarthritic hip or knee, or insoles, to correct shortening or deformity of the legs, may be of tremendous value.

Drugs

Simple analgesics and non-steroidal anti-inflammatory drugs (NSAIDs) are both used extensively for osteoarthritis. It is often appropriate to use them 'on demand', e.g. before gardening or on a day when pain is particularly bad. NSAIDs provide greater symptomatic benefit in many patients than the simple analgesic agents. However, their regular use is associated with a significant incidence of side-effects (*see* p. 37) and short courses are preferable to continuous use. Steroid injections into joints have a limited role, though aspiration of swollen inflamed knee joints and infusion of a long-acting steroid preparation may occasionally provide considerable benefit.

Surgery

Osteotomy provides immediate pain relief and may lead to an improvement in the X-ray changes of the joint concerned. Arthroplasty (prosthetic joint replacement) gives good results in patients with severe pain, resting and night pain, and significant disability. Although mortality rates are low, there is a substantial morbidity associated with prosthetic surgery, especially loosening of the prosthesis and sepsis. Improvements in prosthetic materials and cements are continually being made, which should reduce these problems. Joint fusion or arthrodesis may occasionally be considered, especially if other procedures have failed.

RHEUMATOID ARTHRITIS

Rheumatoid arthritis is a systemic connective-tissue disorder causing predominantly a symmetrical polyarthritis of peripheral synovial joints. It is thought to result from abnormal immunological responses to an unidentified triggering agent (possibly a virus) in genetically susceptible individuals. Both humoral and cell mediated mechanisms are involved.

Clinical features

The joints most commonly involved by rheumatoid arthritis are the proximal interphalangeal joints, metacarpal–phalangeal joints, wrists, metatarsal–phalangeal joints and knees. Involved joints show evidence of active inflammation, i.e. they are hot, painful, especially on movement, with soft tissue swelling and, eventually, bone deformity and destruction. Typical X-ray changes are loss of joint space, juxta-articular osteopenia and bony erosions around the joint margins.

Onset is commonly in middle age, with women being three times more frequently affected than men. It is a chronic condition with a low mortality, so patients frequently live with it into their later years. Subjects who develop rheumatoid arthritis in their early years may either survive into old age with no major disabilities or with considerable joint destruction. However, the disease may arise for the first time in the later decades of life in a substantial proportion of patients, where it has a more benign prognosis. The female preponderance, seen in younger rheumatoid patients, tends to disappear with age, so that men and women are then almost equally affected. Later onset is often abrupt, if not explosive, with a similar distribution of joint involvement as in younger patients. Erosions and nodules are less common than in younger subjects, while rheumatoid arteritis is rare in elderly patients. Tests for rheumatoid factor often show a high titre, but this is not necessarily associated with a poor prognosis. Except for anaemia, extra-articular manifestations, e.g. pulmonary involvement and neuropathy, are uncommon. Though distinct from osteoarthritis, the two conditions may occasionally be seen in the same patient, when deformed, 'burnt out' rheumatoid joints are subject to the degenerative changes of osteoarthritis (Table 11.1).

Table 11.1 *Comparison of radiological features of osteoarthritis and rheumatoid arthritis*

Radiological features	*Osteoarthritis*	*Rheumatoid arthritis*
Joints principally affected	Hip and knee, spine	Hands and feet, wrist (knee, less commonly)
Symmetry of joint involvement	Often asymmetrical	Usually symmetrical
Joint space narrowing	Maximal at weight-bearing sites	Uniform
Erosions	Absent (may be mimicked by degeneration of articular surface)	Present
Density of juxta-articular bone	Increased (subchondral sclerosis)	Decreased (osteopenia)
Osteophytes	Present	Absent

Treatment

The general principles of treatment of elderly patients are similar to those in younger patients, but with minor modifications. Treatment should be directed towards relieving symptoms and improving function by:

1. Maintenance of mobility by physiotherapy.
2. Preventing deformities with splints.
3. Minimizing symptoms with drugs.

Physiotherapy can only be undertaken and benefit achieved if joint pain and discomfort have been sufficiently lessened beforehand. Prolonged bed rest must be avoided in the acute stages of the disease, because of the risk of pressure sores, deep venous thrombosis, etc. Positioning of the patient when in bed to prevent deformity is important, i.e. pillows should not be placed under the knees, whilst supports should be given to the arms and feet. Splintage of inflamed joints, particularly of the knees and wrists, is important to prevent contractures and provides both pain relief and joint support. Joint protection is an essential part of treatment, consisting of providing aids and teaching the patient techniques for avoiding joint strain. Shoes should be comfortable and large enough to allow for any foot deformity. Difficulty in rising from a chair may be overcome by the provision of one of the correct height and shape, although spring-assisted seats may occasionally be necessary.

Drug treatment

NSAIDs (*see* Chapter 4)

These drugs are extremely useful analgesic agents but they are often associated with serious side-effects, especially in elderly patients. Currently there are a bewildering 18 different agents to choose from. Many have been developed to provide efficacy with a low incidence of adverse reactions. Comparative trials have not yet provided any clear picture overall of the relative efficacy of individual members of this large group of drugs. Variation in tolerance is wide and difficult to predict in individual patients. In general, though account should be taken of pharmacokinetic data, the choice of an NSAID for any individual patient rests upon trial and error. Drug treatment for each patient should be designed to give the maximum efficacy with the minimum of side-effects.

Corticosteroids

Oral corticosteroids may cause a dramatic improvement in the arthritis and general well-being of a patient with rheumatoid arthritis, regardless of age. However, prolonged courses of high-dose steroids must be avoided because of the development of long-term complications; elderly subjects, in particular, are prone to develop vertebral collapse, diabetes, psychosis and hypertension. However, small doses, e.g. 7.5 mg of prednisolone, may be justified as they may be sufficient to provide benefit, but with a small likelihood of side-effects. Intra-articular injections of corticosteroids are often extremely beneficial during phases of acute joint inflammation. Care must be taken with patients of any age to avoid introducing infection. Aspiration of synovial fluid beforehand for inspection or bacterial culture is therefore advisable.

Other drug therapies

Gold and *d*-penicillamine may be effective in arresting active disease. Both drugs may cause side-effects and require careful monitoring. They may be used in elderly subjects, but this treatment is best undertaken after specialist rheumatological advice has been sought.

Surgery

Removal of an inflamed synovial membrane of an affected joint without gross destructive change may provide dramatic pain relief. As with patients who have osteoarthritis, arthrodesis and arthroplasty are other treatment options which may provide pain relief and, with arthroplasty, restoration of joint function.

OTHER ARTHROPATHIES

There are many other possible causes of painful joints in elderly patients, as shown in Table 11.2. Their diagnosis and treatment is the same as for younger patients. Crystal synovitis (gout and pseudo-gout) is often seen in elderly subjects, whilst mixed forms of arthritis are not uncommon, e.g. rheumatoid arthritis and septic arthritis.

Table 11.2 *Causes of joint pain in elderly subjects*

Common	*Uncommon*
Osteoarthritis	Systemic sclerosis
Rheumatoid arthritis	Polyarteritis nodosa
Gout	Systemic lupus erythematosus
Pyrophosphate arthropathy (pseudo-gout)	Dermatomyositis
Septic arthritis	
Psoriatic arthritis	

MEDICAL ASPECTS OF HIP SURGERY IN ELDERLY PATIENTS

Fractures of the femoral neck

The incidence of bony fractures increases with increasing age, partly because there is an age-related decline in mechanical strength of bones (i.e. osteoporosis, *see* p. 130), but also because of an increased liability of elderly people to fall, due to poor righting reflexes and a reduction in postural control (*see* p. 96). Common fractures in elderly people are those of the spinal vertebrae, the forearm and femoral neck, of which the last is of particular importance in terms of morbidity and mortality. Fractures in young people usually require direct trauma, whereas older people tend to suffer fractures in the absence of external violence, the majority occurring as a result of falls at home.

Fractures of the neck of the femur carry a substantial overall mortality, occurring three times as often in elderly women as in elderly men. Two major types are recognized:

1. Fractures occurring within the joint capsule, i.e. subcapital and transcervical fractures (approximately 60% of the total fractures). These fractures are associated with a low mortality. Because of the high incidence of bony non-union, replacement of the femoral head by an artificial prosthesis is often required.
2. Fractures occurring outside the joint capsule, i.e. intertrochanteric and subtrochanteric (approximately 40% of the total fractures). These are associated with a higher immediate mortality and require internal fixation and sometimes reduction of the bony fragments. The fractures occur through cancellous bone with a good blood supply and therefore bony union is usually achieved.

Hip replacement surgery

Hip replacement surgery may be performed electively because of painful osteoarthritis, to give relief from pain and stiffness and preserve or increase mobility. In selected cases, it may also be used for end-stage arthritis to make nursing care easier for patient and carers alike, thereby improving patients' quality of life, while also helping to reduce the demand for community health and welfare services. However, it may have to be undertaken as an emergency after certain types of femoral neck fractures.

A strong, biologically inert metal head and neck replaces the femoral head while a high-density plastic cup replaces the bony acetabulum. This combination is designed to produce minimal wear and have a long life. Precise details of the many prostheses available should be sought in specialist orthopaedic texts. These prostheses are held in place by material functioning as cement. Much research is currently under way to improve the physical properties of the available cements.

MEDICAL MANAGEMENT OF THE ELDERLY ORTHOPAEDIC PATIENT

At present in the UK, approximately one in four patients admitted to surgical beds is over 65 years of age and about 10% are over 70 years. In orthopaedic wards, the admission rate almost doubles for each decade after the age of 65 years. Much of the excess morbidity and mortality in the older patient appears to have its roots in coincidental medical problems present at the time of operation, which provides the rationale for a careful pre-operative medical assessment.

The medical management of any elderly patient undergoing surgery, orthopaedic or otherwise, requires an understanding of the likely problems that may arise from diminished physiological reserves and multiple intercurrent pathology. Various studies give mortality figures in patients over 70 years of 5 to 23%. All agree that surgical mortality increases with increasing age and that it is higher after emergency compared with elective surgery.

Pre-operative assessment

Pre-operative assessment of the patients' mental and physical state should be as thorough as possible before surgery. Assessment of *cardiovascular state* is particularly important to ensure that the patient can withstand the stress of surgery. The risk of dying post-operatively is increased by prior evidence of congestive cardiac failure, the presence of cardiac arrhythmias, significant aortic stenosis or a history of myocardial infarction in the previous six months.

The relative pulmonary overinflation and rigidity of the chest wall with advancing age is responsible for a *reduction in the respiratory reserve* of elderly patients. This, together with the frequent occurrence of chronic obstructive airways disease, makes respiratory assessment essential so that any bronchospasm or infection is treated pre-operatively and physiotherapy given to prevent sputum retention.

Salt and water depletion prior to surgery is common in elderly patients, especially if they have been receiving chronic (and often inappropriate) diuretic therapy. If hypovolaemia is not detected pre-operatively, it tends to manifest itself at the time of induction of anaesthesia as a sharp drop in blood pressure, with consequent renal impairment.

Medications, both prescribed and actually taken, must be documented and assessed to determine whether it is necessary to continue them. The potential for harmful drug interactions and the age-related changes in renal and hepatic function must be borne in mind before any fresh drugs are prescribed (*see* Chapter 4).

Pre-operative *anaemia* carries a bad prognostic influence on any surgery. However, unless there has been precipitous blood loss just beforehand, correction of the anaemia will not improve the postoperative outcome. The presence of anaemia pre-operatively is correlated with serious illness and it is this which is responsible for postoperative morbidity and mortality.

There is a close relationship between *nutritional state* and immunological function. Therefore a malnourished surgical patient may be expected to have an increased post-operative incidence of sepsis and perhaps other complications. Time spent improving the nutritional status of a patient before elective surgery is well used.

Postoperative complications

Respiratory

Postoperative respiratory problems in elderly general surgical patients, estimated to be between 20 and 40%, are the most common cause of postoperative death. In the majority of cases, it has been demonstrated that small airways closure is the primary event, resulting in atelectasis and, when infection occurs, pneumonia. However, a minority of patients develop retention of respiratory secretions, resulting in airways blockage and hence atelectasis and pneumonia. Assistance from physiotherapists is therefore important to encourage deep breathing and coughing exercises to keep the airways clear. The time spent by an elderly patient immobile in bed and thus more susceptible to chest infections should be kept to a minimum.

Cardiovascular

The two main complications that occur in elderly patients are myocardial infarction (often painless) and cardiac failure. Risk factors include increasing age, poor exercise tolerance, previous cardiac disease and emergency surgery. In patients with known ischaemic heart disease, the risk is at its highest in the presence of unstable angina or when myocardial infarction has occurred less than six months before operation. *Deep venous thrombosis* is very common after orthopaedic operations and *pulmonary embolism*, not an uncommon cause of death. Many surgeons now use prophylactic subcutaneous heparin pre-operatively to reduce both complications and sometimes post-operatively, until patients regain their mobility.

Confusion

Some degree of disorientation and restlessness is common in old people after anaesthesia. This is usually transient, but if prolonged, an explanation needs to be found so that it can be treated and, hopefully, reversed. Common treatable causes are dehydration and electrolyte disturbances, especially hyponatraemia, hypoxaemia and pain or discomfort from faecal impaction, a full bladder or arthritic joints. Drugs, for instance, anticholinergic drugs, may be responsible for producing acute toxic psychoses. Medical 'events' may occur in the postoperative period, e.g. myocardial infarction or stroke, and may be responsible for the development of acute confusional states. These need to be recognized and treated in their own right.

Stroke

Postoperative strokes occur in about 1% of general surgical patients aged 65 or more, while patients over 80 years have an incidence of about 3%. Autoregulation of the cerebral circulation is impaired with age and therefore it is particularly desirable to avoid extremes of hypotension or hypertension during surgery. A further preventative measure, which lies with the anaesthetist, is careful positioning of the elderly neck, to avoid occlusion of vertebral or carotid arteries.

Pressure sores

These lesions may develop extremely rapidly in elderly patients immobile in bed postoperatively, unless attention is given to pressure areas to prevent them. Similarly, patients are at particular risk preoperatively if kept waiting in accident and emergency departments for long periods on hard trolleys. The development of pressure sores causes much discomfort and sometimes chronic infection, delaying rehabilitation and discharge home. Prevention being preferable to cure, all patients should be assessed for their risk of developing pressure sores and remedial steps taken so that they do not develop them (*see* Chapter 13).

The rehabilitation team

The skills of the multidisciplinary rehabilitation team are particularly valuable in the postoperative care of elderly surgical and orthopaedic patients. The skills of the physiotherapist, occupational therapist, dietician and social worker may all be required to restore these patients to their optimum functional state, either living in their own homes once again or being cared for elsewhere. With modern techniques, most elderly patients tolerate surgery very well and their long-term survival is at least as good as age-matched patients in the general population.

Chapter

12

Common Endocrine Problems

HYPOTHYROIDISM (MYXOEDEMA) • HYPERTHYROIDISM • DIABETES MELLITUS • METABOLIC BONE DISEASE

Elderly people are subject to the same range of endocrine diseases as younger patients. However, thyroid disease, diabetes mellitus and metabolic bone disease occur commonly and will be described in some detail.

HYPOTHYROIDISM (MYXOEDEMA)

Functional activity of the thyroid gland declines with age. There is a wide gradation of declining thyroid activity with increasing age, so that hypothyroidism cannot be considered an 'all or none' phenomenon. During this time, the pituitary gland secretes increasing amounts of thyroid-stimulating hormone (TSH) to stimulate the thyroid, in an attempt to maintain thyroid hormone levels in the normal range. However, once the thyroid reserve has been completely exhausted and no further increase in thyroid hormones can be obtained by increasing concentrations of TSH, clinical evidence of thyroid failure will become apparent.

Causes

The majority of patients have an autoimmune basis for their thyroid failure. Autoimmune thyroiditis may be associated with thyroid atrophy or with the presence of a goitre, as a late manifestation of

Hashimoto's disease. Eighty per cent of patients with hypothyroidism have thyroid autoantibodies, often give a family history of thyroid disease and have evidence of other autoimmune diseases, particularly pernicious anaemia and vitiligo.

Thyroid failure may also be seen in elderly subjects whose thyroid activity has already been reduced by previous treatment for thyrotoxicosis, whether by surgery or radioactive iodine therapy. Hypothyroidism may occasionally occur secondary to hypopituitarism, which may be idiopathic or follow pituitary infarction or destruction by a cerebral tumour (e.g. craniopharyngioma). Features of hypothyroidism may occasionally develop again in a patient previously diagnosed as having myxoedema, if for any reason there is failure in compliance with thyroid replacement.

Clinical features

The classical picture of hypothyroidism is easy to recognize. However, the gradual and insidious slowing of physical and mental functions of hypothyroid patients is often wrongly ascribed to the natural ageing process. Women are affected five times more commonly than men. Elderly people with hypothyroidism may have a non-specific presentation with impaired mobility and declining general health, and are frequently seen as apathetic or depressed. Pain or tingling in the hands may draw attention to the presence of the carpal tunnel syndrome. Constipation is almost universal.

Rarely, hypothyroidism may present with cerebellar ataxia or various psychiatric disturbances, while pleural and pericardial effusions and ascites are occasionally present, but seldom cause symptoms. All these symptoms and signs are reversed with treatment. Hypothyroid patients are more susceptible than normal to hypothermia and are at particular risk if they also take sedative drugs, which themselves are metabolized more slowly than normal. Anaemia, usually normocytic, is present in 30% of patients and reflects the reduced metabolic demand of the hypothyroid state, mediated by reduced levels of erythropoietin.

The well-known clinical sign of hypothyroidism—delayed relaxation of the ankle jerk—may be difficult to obtain in the presence of oedematous feet and ankles. (This tendon reflex is frequently absent in elderly people.) However, delayed relaxation may be demonstrated with other tendon reflexes; the biceps or supinator reflexes may show this feature extremely well.

Diagnosis

The diagnosis of myxoedema is aided by a high index of suspicion and confirmed by an elevated concentration of serum TSH.

Treatment

Hypothyroidism is treated by replacement thyroxine. This must be started as a very small dose (i.e. 25 or 50 μg) and increased at two-weekly intervals, until a maintenance daily dose of 100 to 200 μg is reached. Slow initial replacement is essential to prevent cardiac failure, with or without myocardial infarction. Synthetic thyroxine has a long duration of action, is well absorbed orally and need not be given more than once a day. However, for patients with compliance problems, weekly or twice weekly supervision of thyroxine ingestion by the district nurse may be equally satisfactory.

HYPERTHYROIDISM

Hyperthyroidism is caused by increased secretion by the thyroid gland of either or both thyroxine (T4) and tri-iodothyronine (T3). It used to be thought that hyperthyroidism was uncommon in elderly people. With the increasing size of the elderly population and the growing medical interest in them, this assumption has been proved false, with approximately 20% of all cases being over 70 years old. As with younger patients, women are more frequently affected than men.

Causes

Multinodular goitres predispose towards the development of hyperthyroidism and are the commonest cause of thyroid overactivity. They are common findings at post mortem examinations of elderly people, though they have often been clinically unapparent during life. In contrast, classical Graves' disease with the typical eye signs is relatively rare in the elderly. Occasionally, toxic thyroid adenomas arise, which are 'hot' on a thyroid scintiscan, and secrete thyroid hormones independently of any normal control from the pituitary gland.

Clinical features

The characteristic features of restlessness, tachycardia and heat intolerance in the presence of a diffuse goitre, together with hot, sweaty, trembling hands, are often inconspicuous in older patients, who usually present in a more non-specific way. Indeed, the presentation of thyrotoxicosis may be so different in a small minority of patients as even to suggest underactivity of the thyroid gland. Patients may feel weak, lethargic and depressed or appear wasted, chronically ill or apathetic, giving rise to their having what is called 'masked' or 'apathetic' hyperthyroidism.

Cardiac problems may frequently predominate because the thyroid hormones sensitize the heart to catecholamines, giving rise to a hyperdynamic circulation with an increased heart rate and cardiac output. Hence, symptoms such as palpitations, angina and dyspnoea may arise—but these, of course, commonly occur as a result of ischaemic heart disease as well. However, cardiac failure of obscure origin should always raise this possible aetiology, especially if it is precipitated by a supraventricular tachyarrhythmia. Atrial fibrillation is very common and is resistant to digoxin treatment because the clearance of digoxin is enhanced by the hyperdynamic circulation and blood levels are lower than otherwise expected.

Weight loss may be present with an associated increased appetite or, sometimes, anorexia. It may however be masked by the fluid retention of cardiac failure. Weight loss is always a serious symptom for which many other conditions may be responsible. Diarrhoea is an uncommon presenting symptom of thyrotoxicosis, but an increase in the individual's normal bowel habit is usual. However, when associated with anorexia, nausea and abdominal pain, this change in bowel habit needs to be differentiated from other conditions of gastrointestinal pathology. Such symptoms may closely mimic a colonic neoplasm.

Mental disturbances, such as the rapid onset of confusion or psychoses, are common and may obscure the clinical picture. Generalized muscle wasting may occur, with muscle weakness and consequent falls being a presenting complaint. Thyrotoxic myopathy may be demonstrated by electromyography, with muscles of the limb girdles being principally affected. A fine hand tremor is a classical sign of hyperthyroidism in young patients; tremor is so common in the elderly for other reasons that it is of little significance in making this diagnosis.

Diagnosis

The diagnosis of thyrotoxicosis in elderly patients is often difficult. Clinical suspicions must be confirmed by laboratory data. At the current time, the plasma thyroxine, both total and free forms of the hormone, appears the most reliable investigation, occasionally needing confirmation by very low levels of TSH and a suppressed thyrotrophin-releasing hormone (TRH) test. A thyroid scintiscan may show generalized increased uptake of radioactive iodine, the presence of multinodular activity or a single 'hot' adenoma.

Treatment

Thyroid irradiation using ^{131}I remains the treatment of choice for elderly patients with thyrotoxicosis because of its ease and simplicity. However, this treatment takes two to three months to become effective, and if rapid control is required (e.g. to control cardiac failure), antithyroid drugs may need to be used in addition until this takes effect. Carbimazole is the drug commonly used but, as it may rarely cause agranulocytosis, patients should be warned of the need to seek medical advice if they should develop a fever or other evidence of infection. Beta-receptor blocking drugs, often used in the initial treatment of young thyrotoxic patients, should not be used in elderly patients because of the risk of inducing cardiac failure.

The amount of ^{131}I required to control thyroid overactivity without either the recurrence of the overactive state or the long-term development of hypothyroidism is difficult to calculate with any certainty. It is therefore generally agreed that the thyroid irradiation should aim to ablate the thyroid gland and thus the need for life-long T4 replacement will occur in all patients. However, the presence of a goitre causing pressure symptoms will require surgery, whatever the age of the patient. As mentioned above, such surgery carries a significant risk of subsequent hypothyroidism, in addition to the very small postoperative risks of laryngeal nerve palsy and hypoparathyroidism, with tetany and paraesthesiae.

DIABETES MELLITUS

Diabetes mellitus is common in the elderly population, being found *de novo* in elderly subjects as well as in those in whom the diagnosis has been made in their earlier years. Diabetic complications, affecting the eyes, peripheral nerves, kidneys and arteries, are frequently seen in elderly patients. Some elderly patients require insulin and have insulin-dependent (IDDM) or Type 1 diabetes, whilst the majority have non-insulin dependent diabetes (NIDDM) or Type 2 diabetes. The condition is obvious in the presence of sufficient hyperglycaemia to cause polyuria and polydipsia, resulting from the osmotic diuresis and consequent dehydration. Similarly, a random plasma glucose of 11 mmol/l or more (or alternatively, 10 mmol/l or more in venous whole blood) in symptomatic patients makes a formal glucose tolerance test unnecessary. However, in asymptomatic patients, two or more values above 11 mmol/l are diagnostic.

If symptoms are absent or blood glucose values are equivocal, the diagnostic criteria for diabetes are shown by the blood glucose response to a standard 2-hour 75 g oral glucose tolerance test. Venous plasma glucose concentrations rise from fasting levels of 8 mmol/l or more, to 11 mmol/l or more at two hours after the glucose load (normal values less than 6 mmol/l and less than 8 mmol/l, respectively).

Values between those of the diabetic and normal range are considered to show an impaired glucose tolerance, a feature of increasing age. Several surveys have shown that over 50% of people over 70 years old have such abnormal glucose tolerance curves. These people are at risk of developing large vessel disease, i.e. cerebrovascular, peripheral vascular and coronary artery disease, while a small proportion (about 3% per year) go on to develop overt, symptomatic diabetes. They should not be treated with specific antidiabetic treatment, although obesity may require dietary advice to achieve an appropriate weight loss. Drugs such as the thiazide diuretics and corticosteroids impair glucose tolerance further and may precipitate diabetic symptoms. When this occurs, they must therefore be discontinued wherever possible.

The aim of treatment

The aim of treatment of a young diabetic is to keep blood glucose levels as near the normal range as possible, in the hope of preventing the late microvascular complications of the disease. However, in the older patient, such long-term aims are not applicable and treatment should therefore be designed to:

1. Prevent hyperglycaemic symptoms.
2. Avoid over-zealous treatment leading to hypoglycaemia, which is poorly tolerated in the elderly.
3. Anticipate and minimize decompensation during intercurrent illness.
4. Prevent and manage complications, such as foot ulcers and retinopathy.

Blood glucose levels in elderly diabetics should be tailored to be between 6 and 12 mmol/l—both avoiding the risk of hypoglycaemia and levels of hyperglycaemia that cause symptoms. The renal threshold is variable in the elderly, so the presence of glycosuria is of less value in monitoring glycaemic control than in the younger patient. Over-treatment is always more dangerous than under-treatment. Hypoglycaemia may have an atypical presentation; confusion or focal neurological signs, e.g. a transient hemiparesis, may occur, with possible permanent neurological damage if it is not immediately recognized.

General care

General measures to improve or maintain the health of elderly diabetics include: advice about the maintenance of a normal body weight, the value of gentle exercise, wherever feasible, and control of cardiovascular risk factors (e.g. hypertension and smoking). Advice about foot care is most important to avoid the development of ulcers. If patients cannot look after their own feet, regular chiropody should be arranged.

Screening for visual impairment and the detection of treatable diabetic retinopathy should be undertaken at regular intervals so that vision is preserved for as long as possible. This is of particular importance to insulin-requiring diabetics, whose poor sight may cause difficulty with their injections.

Patients and their relatives should be warned of the risks of further impairment of glucose tolerance in the event of episodes of infection, stress or minor surgery and advised of the necessity to seek medical attention immediately.

Dietary advice

Dietary advice is essential both for diabetics requiring tablets or insulin and also for asymptomatic diabetic elderly patients, for whom it is likely to be their sole mode of treatment. It should be simple and easily understood; refined sugar should be avoided, with starch- and high fibre-containing foods taken in its place. The obese should be encouraged to lose weight. The help of a dietician is of great value to provide detailed advice and also information about the nutritional status of commonly eaten foods. However, dietary restrictions and alterations of life-style should not be made at the expense of patients' quality of life.

Oral hypoglycaemic drugs

Oral hypoglycaemic drugs are used if dietary advice is insufficient to relieve symptoms of hyperglycaemia. The *sulphonylureas* act by increasing the secretion of insulin from the pancreas. They are highly bound to plasma proteins and are metabolized by the liver and the metabolites excreted by the kidneys. The long duration of action of chlorpropamide (half-life in young patients of 24–60 hours) makes it a dangerous drug in the elderly, who are susceptible to its prolonged hypoglycaemic effects. It may frequently be associated with troublesome nocturnal hypoglycaemic episodes as well as focal neurological deficits, and should therefore not be used. Gliclazide, with a half-life of 10–12 hours may be given as a single morning dose, while tolbutamide, acting for 6–8 hours, is also a useful drug in elderly patients, being given twice or three times each day.

Metformin is the only *biguanide* now available in the UK, and may help in some obese diabetic patients. Its short half-life of 6 hours makes it less likely to cause hypoglycaemia than the sulphonylureas. It acts by increasing peripheral utilization of glucose and is excreted largely unchanged by the kidneys. It rarely causes lactic acidosis, usually in the presence of other serious disease, e.g. cardiac failure, hypoxia or severe renal impairment.

Insulin

Insulin treatment is necessary in those patients who have developed diabetic ketoacidosis and in those whose symptoms are not controlled by diet and tablets. It may also be required temporarily in patients rendered hyperglycaemic by acute infections or acute stress (e.g. after a myocardial infarct, stroke or while undergoing surgery), as well as in the initial treatment of hyperosmolar non-ketotic coma.

Most elderly patients can be managed by once daily injections, which patients themselves prefer, or if they cannot give their own injections, can be manageable for district nurses to give. Hypoglycaemia should be avoided at all costs, especially if the patients live alone, where episodes of confusion or coma can be dangerous or even life-threatening. It is particularly important to emphasize to all patients on insulin therapy the need for a bedtime snack to avoid nocturnal hypoglycaemia.

HYPEROSMOLAR NON-KETOTIC COMA

Some 10 to 20% of patients whose diabetes presents with hyperglycaemic coma do not have marked ketoacidosis. Such patients are usually middle-aged or elderly and many may not previously be known to be diabetic. The history, which may be gradual or sudden, is of increasing weakness, drowsiness and confusion, which may lead to coma. There may be a history of thirst and polyuria, often associated with drinking high-carbohydrate drinks, such as Lucozade. The level of consciousness is directly related to the degree of hyperosmolarity. Focal neurological signs may occur and fits develop in 25% of patients.

These patients have severe dehydration and hypotension, as a result of their marked osmotic diuresis. Biochemical abnormalities include extreme hyperglycaemia (greater than 50 mmol/l) and hypernatraemia, but ketone bodies are absent from the blood and the pH is normal. Treatment consists of replacement of lost fluid with saline (which should be isotonic if the plasma sodium is below 150 mmol/l, but half normal otherwise) and insulin. The mortality is high with rates of 40 to 50% being reported, but those who recover can often be managed long-term without insulin, by dietary control and oral hypoglycaemic drugs.

METABOLIC BONE DISEASE

Metabolic bone diseases typically affect the whole skeleton. The two common forms in old age are osteoporosis and osteomalacia and as with many diseases of the elderly, they may exist together. Paget's disease, a disease which predominantly affects the elderly population, will also be described.

Osteoporosis

Osteoporosis (or osteopenia) describes the condition where there is a reduction in the total amount of skeletal bone. There is a slow, progressive loss of bone which occurs with increasing age. As women have lighter skeletons than men, this age-related loss is of greater significance to women, whose bones more readily reach a critically thin stage at which symptoms occur. Such osteoporotic bone is histologically normal and measurements of serum calcium, phosphorus and alkaline phosphatase are all within the normal range.

Postmenopausal (type 1) osteoporosis is said to affect women up to the age of 70 and is characterized by predominantly trabecular bone loss leading to vertebral fractures. *'Senile' (type 2) osteoporosis* usually affects people over 75; cortical and trabecular bone are lost equally and fractures of the femur are characteristic.

Secondary osteoporosis often follows from excess levels of adrenal corticosteroids, either in endogenous form, as in Cushing's syndrome, or where they are used as drug therapy for rheumatoid arthritis, asthma or skin diseases. Malignancy, especially myeloma, thyrotoxicosis, chronic liver disease and alcoholism, all cause accelerated bone loss.

There is evidence to suggest that the amount of bone in old age is determined by the maximum achieved at skeletal maturity. Skeletal development may be influenced by many factors: physical activity, disease, nutrition, and by endocrine and racial factors. Women have poorer skeletal development compared with men and for a decade around the menopause, lose bone rapidly as a consequence of oestrogen deficiency. Elderly women therefore have lighter skeletal masses and are more likely to develop bone pain and fractures than men.

Immobilization, from prolonged bed rest, causes (or worsens) generalized osteoporosis, whereas immobility, caused by a fracture, joint disease or hemiplegia, leads to more localized osteoporosis. The importance of nutritional factors, especially calcium deficiency, is an area of much controversy. At present it seems that they do not have a major role in the aetiology of osteoporosis.

Clinical features

Osteoporosis is a condition predominately affecting elderly women. It may be completely asymptomatic; when associated with symptoms, the spine is the area usually affected earliest and most severely. The cardinal feature of osteoporosis is backache of the lower dorsal/upper lumbar spine, occasionally radiating to the buttocks and down the legs. The pain is relieved by lying flat and aggravated by movement. Girdle pain from nerve root compression is rare. Symptoms are often intermittent, occurring for no obvious reason.

Crush or compression fractures of one or more dorsal or lumbar vertebrae are often found, which are responsible for a progressive loss of height. The vertebrae are not uniformly involved. The onset of such fractures may or may not be heralded by pain. Loss of height due to shortening of the trunk may be seen as a dorsal kyphosis develops: the crown–pubis distance become progressively less than the pubis–heel distance. In severe cases, the lower ribs may override the iliac crests. Osteoporosis predisposes to fracture of other bones after a fall or minimal trauma. Fractures of the neck of the femur, pubic rami, forearm and upper end of the humerus are common in elderly women.

Though levels of alkaline phosphatase are usually in the normal range, a moderate rise in the alkaline phosphatase is seen for a month or more after a fracture, reflecting reparative osteoblastic activity.

X-ray changes

The radiological hallmark of osteoporosis is an increased translucency of bone. This affects all bones, but particularly the trabecular bone of the spine. Radiological rarefaction of bone presents problems in accurate standardization, as bone appearances are markedly affected by radiographic exposure factors. To quantify bone density, single and dual photon absorptiometry and quantitative computerized tomography are now becoming more freely available and may improve this situation in the future. Bodies of the lumbar vertebrae become biconcave in appearance, because of the expansion into them of the intervertebral discs. Crush fractures are seen as reduced height of the vertebral bodies, with wedging on the lateral views where the narrower ends are directed internally. A reduction in cortical thickness is found in osteoporotic long bones.

Prevention and treatment

Current research centres around the prevention of osteoporosis. At the menopause, there is an accelerated loss of bone, which can be diminished by oestrogen treatment. The negative calcium balance exhibited by menopausal women is reduced with oestrogen therapy and postmenopausal women who have had this treatment are known to develop fewer bone fractures than those who have not. However, this treatment has not been used with very elderly women because of the vaginal bleeding and psychological upset which it would cause. Whether oestrogen therapy would be as effective as in younger women remains unknown. Other studies have shown conflicting results from the administration of various combinations of calcium supplements, fluoride supplements and vitamin D.

Treatment of established osteoporosis remains problematical, although an adequate calcium intake in the diet seems a reasonable first step. In elderly patients, symptoms are often episodic, relating to the appearance of crush fractures, and may themselves be self-limiting. When present, pain should be relieved by analgesics, while muscular support to the bones can often be improved by exercises from the physiotherapist. Occasionally, the temporary use of a lumbosacral support to the spine or a walking stick may be necessary to enable a patient to remain physically active. As with many conditions, prevention is better than cure and immobilization of elderly people, whether sick or well, should be avoided wherever possible.

Most patients with osteoporosis remain well with their life expectancy little affected by it. However, two conditions related to osteoporosis directly threaten life: long-bone fractures, especially of the femoral neck, carry a significant mortality, while the diminution of vital capacity of the lungs caused by shortening and kyphosis of the thoracic spine may be deleterious if patients develop pneumonia.

Osteomalacia

Osteomalacia is a generalized disease of bone characterized by inadequate calcification of the bone matrix. It is the adult equivalent of rickets of childhood, caused by deficiency of vitamin D or its metabolites. The bone mass is less strong than normal so that pain is caused on pressure; skeletal deformities and pathological fractures are produced. Its incidence is about 4% in the elderly population admitted to hospital in the UK, with women being more often affected than men. The deficiency of fat-soluble vitamin D may be caused by:

1. Dietary deficiency (*see* p. 42).
2. Malabsorption, e.g. biliary obstruction causing steatorrhoea, jejenal diverticulosis causing the stagnant loop syndrome, coeliac disease, intestinal ischaemia, previous partial gastrectomy (*see* p. 43).
3. Inadequate exposure of the skin to sunlight (NB 10% of the elderly population are housebound).
4. Impaired metabolism of vitamin D, due to liver or renal disease.
5. Drugs affecting vitamin D absorption and metabolism, e.g. liquid paraffin, some anticonvulsants.

Clinical features

Patients with osteomalacia complain of generalized and inconstant muscle pains, especially backache, with muscle weakness and stiffness. They have a specific myopathy of the proximal limb girdles, such that they may have difficulty climbing stairs or getting out of a chair. When severe, the myopathy causes a typical waddling gait. Their bones may be tender on pressure and cause pain on weight bearing. Because they are softer than normal, the bones bend to produce skeletal deformities of the pelvis, increased angulation of the femoral necks and kyphosis. Pathological fractures are also common.

Serum biochemical abnormalities occur with serum calcium concentrations being low or normal, inorganic phosphorus low and alkaline phosphatase high. In considering the serum calcium, it is always advisable to look at the serum albumin at the same time, so that the 'corrected calcium' value can be calculated. The diagnosis of osteomalacia is confirmed by bone biopsy, though this is seldom necessary. Undecalcified bone sections typically show wide uncalcified seams of osteoid bone formation.

X-ray changes

The bones are less dense than normal with thinning of the trabeculae and cortex. Deformities may be seen in the softened bones, with the vertebral bodies being most often affected. On lateral views, they are seen to have become biconcave on their upper and lower surfaces.

(Crush fractures of vertebrae are not typical, though osteoporosis may also be present.) A characteristic finding, not always present, is the appearance of Looser's zones or pseudo-fractures. These are short lucent bands at right angles to the bone cortex, usually extending only part way across the bone. They may have a sclerotic margin, making them more obvious. Common sites for Looser's zones are the pubic rami, axillary border of the scapula and near the lesser trochanter of the femoral head.

Treatment

Once the diagnosis is made, osteomalacia is easily treated. The precise cause of vitamin D deficiency should be established. This may require separate treatment in addition to replacement vitamin D, e.g. a gluten-free diet for coeliac disease or stopping the ingestion of liquid paraffin, thus promoting the absorption of vitamin D. If the diagnosis of osteomalacia is in doubt, a therapeutic trial with vitamin D may be helpful to confirm the presence of osteomalacia. Vitamin D, in the form of oral calciferol, should be given (0.025–0.125 mg or 1000–5000 U daily) for one to three months. As this may produce hypocalcaemia initially, it is usual to give calcium supplements in addition, monitoring the serum calcium closely.

This treatment produces striking symptomatic improvement with rapid disappearance of muscle weakness and bone pain; serum calcium and inorganic phosphate return to normal values. However, the bones take several months to recalcify, with healing of Looser's zones and gradual fall of alkaline phosphatase levels to normal.

Paget's disease (osteitis deformans)

Paget's disease is a progressive disease of bone which affects 5% of the elderly population. It is primarily a disease affecting osteoclasts, such that there is a greatly increased rate of bone remodelling with the formation of structurally abnormal bone. It is a patchy disease: one bone or several may be affected, but unlike osteoporosis and osteomalacia, it is never generalized throughout the skeleton. The affected bone is weak and, at points of stress, becomes deformed with an increased fracture rate. Any bone may be affected; the pelvic girdle, tibia and skull are the most frequently involved. The aetiology of Paget's disease is unknown. Epidemiological data suggest an environmental factor is involved, while there is some cytochemical evidence implicating a slow virus infection.

Clinical features

Paget's disease may be asymptomatic, being discovered by chance on X-ray, or on biochemical screening when high levels of serum alkaline phosphatase are found in the presence of normal serum calcium and phosphate levels. X-rays of the affected bones show that they are thickened and often bowed, with a distorted trabecular pattern and patches of sclerosis and rarefaction. However, there may be pain and deformity of the affected bones, associated with fractures.

Bone enlargement and deformity may be obvious when there is a bowed, thickened tibia; bone distortion may also produce neurological compression. Deafness may result from pressure effects in the bony canals of the auditory apparatus within the skull. Immobilization of affected bone may produce hypercalcaemia, while its increased vascularity may occasionally be sufficiently marked to induce the development of cardiac failure. Rarely, sarcomatous change develops in affected bones.

Treatment

Treatment of bone pain by simple analgesics may be the only therapy required, and should certainly always be tried initially. It may be difficult to distinguish between pain arising from an area of Paget's disease within a bone from pain arising from osteoarthritic change in adjacent joints. There is no evidence at present to suggest that early treatment of the disease prevents progression of long-term complications.

Salmon calcitonin, administered parenterally, improves many of the clinical features of the disease but has a transient suppressive rather than curative effect on bone. Recently, much interest has centred on the use of the orally active diphosphonates. With their high affinity for calcium phosphate crystals, they are powerful inhibitors of crystal formation and dissolution. Pain is frequently relieved and this may persist for a considerable time after treatment has been stopped. Continuous treatment with diphosphonates impairs bone mineralization, therefore intermittent periods of treatment may be needed for maximum pain relief and the formation of structurally normal bone.

Chapter 13

Incontinence and Pressure Sores

URINARY INCONTINENCE • FAECAL INCONTINENCE • CONSTIPATION • PRESSURE SORES

Incontinence and pressure sores are both conditions which may frequently develop in elderly people who are ill. By understanding their aetiology, they can often be completely removed by careful medical and nursing treatment, or even prevented.

URINARY INCONTINENCE

Incontinence, i.e. the involuntary passage of urine, is not a normal accompaniment of old age, although its prevalence rises with increasing age. Approximately 20% of women and 12% of men over 65 years old have some degree of incontinence. It is one of the most important presenting symptoms of illness in the elderly and may be the single most important factor in deciding whether an elderly person can continue living at home. It is not only unpleasant for the sufferers but also for those who live with and care for them. The embarrassment caused by it may frequently be responsible for much social isolation of both patient and family. There are many reasons for incontinence and it is important to establish its cause, as in many cases continence can, with appropriate treatment, be regained.

Physiology of continence and micturition

Continence and the physiology of micturition are complex mechanisms, best described in specialist texts. However, a brief description is necessary to understand how incontinence may develop. Neurological control of bladder function arises at a number of levels and may be understood by considering the development of continence in an infant. As the bladder continually fills with urine from the kidneys, its smooth muscle fibres become distended and stretch receptors are stimulated. This activates the afferent autonomic nerves to the second, third and fourth sacral segments of the spinal cord so that various reflex pathways are activated. These result in parasympathetic (cholinergic muscarinic) efferent nerves being stimulated, which are responsible for producing intrinsic contractions of the bladder. As the bladder becomes more distended, these contractions become more frequent until a large contraction causes the bladder to empty. As time goes by, the child learns to appreciate the sensation of bladder fullness and the social desirability of deciding when and where it is emptied. Thus sensory pathways to the cortex are developed. These pass up the spinal cord to an area in the frontal cerebral cortex within the cingulate gyrus. In addition, there are inhibitory pathways, which pass down the cord to block the reflex arc at the 'sacral bladder centre'. The intrinsic bladder contractions are completely inhibited by the cerebral cortex, but when micturition is consciously desired, this inhibition is lifted. At the same time, striated muscle fibres of the pelvic diaphragm and muscle fibres of the bladder neck and internal sphincter (richly supplied by excitatory adrenergic α-receptors) are relaxed and the bladder is allowed to empty.

Anatomical considerations

The bladder lies on the pelvic diaphragm such that the outlet is normally maintained at a right angle to the urethra. This relationship, essential for continence, is brought about both by the tone of the muscles of the pelvic diaphragm (pubococcygeus and levator ani muscles) and the firm supporting connective tissue surrounding the origin of the urethra, i.e. the internal urethral sphincter. If these tissues are damaged or distorted anatomically (e.g. by a uterine prolapse or cystocoele), the bladder outlet is altered to take on a funnel-like arrangement, as for the initiation of normal micturition. Because of this, after a small rise in abdominal pressure, some urine may leak involuntarily from the bladder.

The urethra is lined by stratified squamous epithelium; the bladder by transitional epithelium. However, the trigone area in women is usually covered by oestrogen-sensitive squamous epithelium. Elderly women frequently develop, because of lack of oestrogens, atrophic changes in the vagina, urethra and trigone that may produce urinary symptoms. Elderly men frequently develop prostatic hypertrophy causing bladder neck obstruction, which may lead to chronic urinary retention with overflow incontinence. Constipation and faecal impaction in both sexes can produce a functional obstruction of the urethra, with the development of urinary retention and incontinence, or alter the urethrovesical angle, as described above to produce incontinence.

Types of incontinence

Stress incontinence

Stress incontinence describes the involuntary leakage of small quantities of urine associated with coughing, sneezing or laughing, or if severe, with any movement. It is associated with the presence of a weak pelvic floor and/or an altered vesical-ureteric angle, often related to childbirth. Vaginal examination will demonstrate the presence of a uterine prolapse or cystocoele, often with the passage of a small quantity of urine visible, on asking the patient to cough or strain. It may be treated by the use of a pessary or gynaecological surgery. For patients who are able to cooperate and who have a small defect, some benefit may be achieved by electrical stimulation (Faradism) or physiotherapy, where the musculature is strengthened by pelvic floor exercises.

Detrusor instability ('unstable bladder')

Any patient with incomplete control of micturition may be said to have an unstable bladder. However, this term is generally used to describe conditions where inadequately suppressed intrinsic contractions of the detrusor muscle occur as a response to bladder filling or other provocative stimuli, such as coughing, laughing or simply changing position. The result is the *total* emptying of the bladder (rather than the small leakage of stress incontinence). It may occur in association with pelvic pathology or without it, and is the commonest cause of incontinence in elderly women and the second commonest cause in elderly men, giving rise to symptoms of frequency, nocturia, urgency and urge incontinence. In many cases, it would seem that the process of cortical inhibition is precariously maintained.

Detrusor instability often responds well to a combination of behavioural therapy for bladder re-training, i.e. improving cortical control by encouraging micturition at defined intervals, and drug treatment to decrease bladder irritability. Drugs with anticholinergic properties, e.g. terodiline, probantheline and the tricyclic antidepressants, will often inhibit minor bladder contractions and restore continence. However, the very high placebo response seen in many instances in drug trials adds weight to its being a functional disorder.

Neurogenic forms of incontinence

The impairment of neurological control of micturition is an important cause of permanent incontinence, and when severe many only be managed by permanent catheterization. The neurological control can be interrupted at several levels as follows.

1. *Loss of cerebral inhibition* may occur with lesions of the cerebral cortex, e.g. stroke (where it may be temporary or permanent), frontal lobe neoplasm or normal pressure hydrocephalus. Patients with Parkinsonism or dementia may also have this form of incontinence, having lost the ability to recognize the implications of the sensation of bladder distension. Forward planning to realize their need for a lavatory and their ability to find it may be grossly impaired, hence urgency and incontinence often results.
2. *Lesions of the spinal cord*, such as damage by trauma, disc prolapse, multiple sclerosis, etc., may interrupt the afferent and efferent pathways from the bladder to higher centres. The sensation of bladder distension is lost, as is the ability to inhibit intrinsic bladder contractions. This results in the typical small volume paraplegic bladder, which empties reflexly under control of the sacral bladder reflex centre. However, emptying is impaired due to diminished or absent coordination between the detrusor and urethral muscles, leaving a residual amount of urine in the bladder, a source of repeated urinary infections. Incoordination may also produce a functional obstruction at the bladder neck, which eventually gives rise to trabeculation and diverticula formation.

3. *Lesions of the cauda equina* may occur with pelvic malignancy, high lumbar disc prolapses and after pelvic surgery. There is an absence of bladder sensation with dribbling incontinence, while examination reveals a considerable volume of residual urine present and peri-anal numbness.
4. *Loss of bladder sensation*: if sensation of bladder distension is lost because of destruction of the afferent sensory fibres but cortical voluntary inhibition retained, the bladder may become greatly distended, producing chronic urinary retention with eventual overflow incontinence. Diseases affecting the posterior nerve roots or posterior horn cells, such as diabetes and tabes dorsalis, may thus be responsible for incontinence. In the early stages, bladder emptying is inadequate with some urine remaining there all the time. This 'residual urine' is therefore an excellent nidus for bacteria to multiply, hence repeated urinary infections occur and these may be responsible for deteriorating renal function.

Investigation of urinary incontinence

Incontinence is a common non-specific presenting symptom of disease in elderly patients, which may be temporary or permanent. Its treatment must be specifically directed to the cause of the incontinence (Table 13.1).

Table 13.1 *Causes of urinary incontinence*

Temporary	Environmental change
	Acute confusional state
	Acute urinary tract infection
	Constipation
	Increased urine volume
	Drugs
Established	Disorders of urethra and pelvic diaphragm (senile vaginitis, urethral prolapse, prostatism, stress incontinence)
	Disorders of bladder (carcinoma, stones, unstable bladder)
	Disorders of neurological control

Temporary incontinence

Before concentrating on specific investigations for incontinence, it is mandatory to examine the patient as a whole, as there are many totally reversible causes of temporary incontinence. Elderly people generally have a neurologically less efficient ability to inhibit micturition and hence continence is more precarious. They therefore suffer a degree of urgency and nocturnal frequency as part of the normal ageing process.

1. *Environmental change*
   Incontinence may be precipitated simply by moving an elderly person into a totally strange environment, like a hospital, where the location of the lavatories may not be known or remembered. Similarly, a poorly mobile patient may be continent at home with a commode nearby, but is rendered incontinent in hospital by not being able to manage the distance from the bed to the lavatory in sufficient time.
2. *Acute confusional states*
   Patients who are acutely confused as a result of, for example, a chest infection or myocardial infarct, may equally become incontinent. Patients who are over-sedated or taking drugs that produce mental confusion may lose the appreciation of bladder sensation and therefore become incontinent.
3. *Urinary infection*
   The urinary frequency and dysuria of an acute urinary tract infection may be associated with a recent onset of incontinence, possibly due to the development of urge incontinence. Treatment usually leads to restoration of continence. However, in many instances of long-standing incontinence, infection is secondary, with treatment having no effect on bladder control. In such cases, therefore, treatment should be directed whenever possible to the cause of the incontinence.
4. *Constipation*
   Constipation and faecal impaction are frequent causes of urinary incontinence (and also of faecal incontinence; *see* p. 145); both are simple to correct. However, it is more helpful to patients to prevent their occurrence. This requires attention both to diet and medication.
5. *Increased urine volume*
   Any cause of diuresis may, by producing rapid bladder filling,

overcome the normal control of its emptying, especially where this is impaired by age or disease. Hyperglycaemia and hypercalcaemia typically produce polyuria and may thus be associated with incontinence; their treatment alone will often restore continence.

6. *Drugs*

   There are numerous drugs that may cause incontinence in elderly subjects. Rapidly acting diuretics producing a brisk diuresis may do so, especially in patients with reduced mobility. Drugs with anticholinergic properties, e.g. tricyclic antidepressants and some drugs used in the treatment of Parkinson's disease, will often cause urinary retention and overflow incontinence by inhibiting parasympathetic nerves to the bladder. Alpha-adrenergic blockade (e.g. by prazocin) will reduce urethral tone and may cause incontinence. In contrast, sympathomimetic bronchodilators, e.g. ephedrine, may produce urinary retention by stimulating the smooth muscle of the urethra, thereby increasing the urethral closing pressure. If drug therapy is responsible for incontinence, efforts must be made either to discontinue the medication or change to alternatives with similar clinical efficacy but different pharmacological properties.

Established incontinence

Before management of established incontinence is attempted, a firm diagnosis of its cause must be made. As part of the history, the number of micturitions during the night and the frequency of micturition by day need to be recorded. Also the presence of dysuria, urgency, dribbling and awareness of bladder distension are important. The nature of any incontinence (*see* above) and its precipitating events are also important. It may be helpful to use an *incontinence chart* whereby normal micturition or incontinence are recorded throughout the day, together with the quantity of liquid consumed. By directing the attention of the patient and family carers or nursing staff to urinary function at regular intervals, some improvement may often be gained. For example, the interval between bladder emptying can be established and the patient encouraged to void before the next involuntary voiding is expected.

Incontinent patients may understandably limit their fluid intake severely. Such a chart may highlight this and an adequate fluid intake be restored, both for general needs and to combat urinary infection. However, for those patients who are incontinent during the night, it is prudent to restrict their fluid intake so that large drinks are not consumed within two to three hours of going to bed.

Physical examination may reveal a palpable bladder or evidence of neurological dysfunction. Rectal examination and vaginal and vulval inspection are essential to demonstrate causes of obstruction or defects in the pelvic diaphragm. Examination of the urine may show infection or haematuria, pointing the way to further investigations that may reveal the presence of bladder calculi or malignancy. Treatment should then be directed towards these specific problems with, hopefully, subsequent resolution of the incontinence.

Specific investigations of continence and bladder function

Cystometry

Cystometry is a useful method of investigating bladder function whereby pressure changes are measured as the bladder is gradually filled. The reaction to increasing distension and to certain provocative stimuli, e.g. coughing, can be observed. Bladder capacity, residual urine volume and the presence or absence of uninhibited bladder contractions can all be measured. Bladder sensation can also be assessed and the volume recorded at which the desire to void is first felt. The urine flow rate may also be recorded. Cystometry can help distinguish between various forms of incontinence, especially those due to stress incontinence, detrusor instability and an uninhibited neurogenic bladder.

Micturating cysto-urethrography

Micturating cysto-urethrography is available in specialist centres. The bladder is filled with a radio-opaque fluid and its shape and any changes in it and in urethral flow are recorded during micturition and demonstrated radiologically. Anatomical abnormalities, e.g. bladder outlet obstruction, which may be structural or functional in origin, as well as pathological conditions of the bladder, such as calculi or carcinoma, can easily be demonstrated.

Cystoscopy

Cystoscopy is generally undertaken by surgeons and reserved for patients in whom specific bladder pathology is suspected. Calculi, bladder papillomata and urethral caruncles can be completely removed. Prostatic enlargement causing bladder obstruction can often be resected at the time of cystoscopy.

Management of established urinary incontinence

If continence cannot be restored, steps should be taken to make the incontinence manageable as far as possible by the patients themselves, or those caring for them by the use of various aids and appliances:

Pad and pants. Incontinence pads may be used while in bed, to offer some protection to the bed linen and reduce laundry problems. Small volumes of urine are adsorbed leaving the surface of the pad and hence the adjacent skin dry. Their capacity is limited, but they are cheap and disposable. For ambulant patients, there are pads available that are worn like a sanitary towel and have at their centre powdered methyl cellulose, which adsorbs urine to form a gel. They can be worn in a special pair of closely fitting pants that have a marsupial pouch in the front where they can be inserted. The pants keep the pads in place but separate them from the skin by a layer of non-wettable polyurethane mesh.

Drainage systems. Various appliances serve to channel and contain the urine but are only successfully used in men. Sheath drainage systems, e.g. Paul's tubing, are worn over the penis and lead by rubber tubing into a drainage bag attached to one leg. The penis needs to be of sufficient length to be suitable for such appliances, which are often extremely useful for cooperative patients. However, they are not suitable for confused patients who may tamper with them or pull them off.

Catheters. Permanent indwelling silastic catheters may often be the only practical solution for incontinence. They channel the urine from the bladder into a polythene bag, which can be attached to the leg or suspended from the waist band thus allowing independence. These bags should contain a flutter valve to prevent backflow so that they may also be worn when the patient is lying in bed. Patients can often be taught to empty the bags themselves every four to six hours. Catheters carry an appreciable risk of added morbidity from urinary infection and may block or be by-passed. They require careful supervision, bladder wash-outs if blocked, and regular changes. Antibiotics should only be used for an acute symptomatic infection, as bacteriuria is always present. Permanent catheterization may represent the only way an incontinent patient can manage at home, in which case the risks are more than counter-balanced by the benefits.

Management of neurogenic incontinence

Where incontinence is due to impaired neurological control, regaining continence may often not be achieved. If there is permanent loss of cerebral inhibition of micturition, continence may sometimes be regained (but usually incontinence only minimized) by regular toileting of the patient. With lesions of the spinal cord and of the cauda equina, there is often a large residual urine volume and permanent catheterization must be considered. (Younger patients with spinal injury may be taught various manoeuvres to empty the bladder manually, or sometimes intermittent self-catheterization, but these methods are seldom appropriate for elderly patients.)

Where there is loss of bladder sensation, encouragement of patients to pass urine voluntarily at regular intervals may prevent bladder distension, at least initially. As some power of voluntary micturition remains, cholinergic drugs, e.g. bethanechol, or drugs that inhibit anticholinesterase, e.g. distigmine, may occasionally be helpful in promoting bladder emptying, as long as side-effects (nausea, blurred vision, bradycardia or intestinal colic) are not too troublesome.

FAECAL INCONTINENCE

Causes (Table 13.2)

As with urinary incontinence, a careful history and examination will usually reveal the cause of faecal incontinence. The involuntary passage of formed stool once or twice a day is most likely to have a neurogenic cause, whereas frequent semi-formed faeces suggests underlying gastrointestinal disease. Constant liquid soiling is usually a consequence of severe constipation with faecal impaction and overflow. This should be readily discovered during the physical examination. Fortunately with correct disgnosis and treatment, faecal incontinence is usually completely preventable.

Table 13.2 *Causes of faecal incontinence*

Diarrhoea due to
—drugs
—gastrointestinal disease
—endocrine disease
Neurogenic
Constipation

Incontinence caused by diarrhoea

Diarrhoea may be associated with faecal incontinence at any age, but especially in the elderly, with their age-related decline in sphincter control and frequent diminished powers of mobility. Drugs are a frequent cause of diarrhoea. Many elderly people continue their lifelong habit of regular purgation, but drugs such as antibiotics may also be implicated.

Disorders of the gastrointestinal tract, such as carcinoma, diverticular disease, ulcerative colitis, proctitis, ischaemic colitis and gastroenteritis, may all cause diarrhoea. Such conditions require investigation and the appropriate treatment. A prolapsed rectum or disrupted anal sphincter due to incomplete haemorrhoid surgery may be responsible for impaired sphincter control and require surgical correction.

Endocrine causes of diarrhoea and associated incontinence include diabetes mellitus and thyrotoxicosis. Diabetic patients may develop diarrhoea as part of the symptom complex of autonomic neuropathy, which may be very resistant to any form of treatment. The diarrhoea of thyrotoxicosis is abolished when the patient is rendered euthyroid.

Neurogenic causes

Incontinence of soft, well-formed faeces may occasionally be found in patients with diffuse cerebrovascular disease, particularly dementia. In such patients, mass bowel movement following the gastro-colic reflex is associated with uninhibited rectal contractions and the passage of normal stools. Often such incontinence is predictable and toileting after meals may remove the problem. Otherwise, it is best to use constipating agents, together with periodic planned evacuation.

CONSTIPATION

Constipation is common in the elderly population and may be aggravated by poor diet, immobility and acute illness. It may be the sinister harbinger of gastrointestinal obstruction and malignancy. Painful anal conditions, e.g. anal fissure and thrombosed haemorrhoids, will also cause constipation. It may be a presenting feature of hypothyroidism, depression and diseases producing hypercalcaemia. Drugs with anticholinergic properties and the opiate analgesics may precipitate severe constipation in patients who already have sluggish bowel function. Diuretics, by causing dehydration and hypokalaemia, may also cause constipation.

Treatment of constipation is ideally directed to its cause. The presence of multiple pathologies, which are almost invariably found in an elderly patient with constipation, must be considered before deciding to embark on specific investigations. A patient with dementia, for example, is unlikely to be able to understand or cooperate in having a barium enema examination and is even less likely to be considered a candidate for major abdominal surgery. However, if no specific cause is found, symptomatic measures should be used.

Laxatives

Laxatives may be administered orally or per rectum (as suppositories or enemas). There are three main categories of laxatives:

1. *Bulking agents*, e.g. bran, ispaghula husk and methylcellulose, which both retain water and promote microbial growth, thereby increasing faecal mass and stimulating peristalsis. A plentiful fluid intake is required. They have very few unwanted side effects.
2. *Osmotic laxatives*, e.g. lactulose, magnesium hydroxide mixture, and magnesium sulphate, which draw fluid into the bowel lumen, thus increasing faecal mass and stimulating peristalsis. As with bulking agents, a plentiful fluid intake is required. However, intestinal cramps may be produced, and in patients with poor

renal function there is the risk of hypermagnesaemia with magnesium-containing agents.

3. *Stimulant laxatives*, e.g. senna, bisacodyl, danthron and docusate preparations, directly stimulate bowel motility and peristalsis. They are effective but may cause intestinal cramps.

After constipation has been cleared, preventative steps should be taken to avoid its recurrence. A high residue diet and adequate fluid intake should be encouraged, while any improvement in mobility will, wherever possible, also be of benefit in the future.

Faecal impaction, overflow diarrhoea and incontinence

When constipation is particularly severe, faeces in the lower colon and rectum gradually becomes more and more dehydrated and hardened, as bowel motility becomes more and more ineffectual. The colonic mucosa becomes irritated and mucus production is stimulated. In addition, the semiliquid faeces at the proximal end of the obstructing mass trickles past, joining the mucus and out through the anus.

Repeated enemas are required to soften and remove the faecal obstruction, after which, preventative measures (e.g. high fibre preparations and maintenance of normal hydration) should be taken to avoid recurrence. Occasionally, manual removal is required initially, a procedure which is unpleasant for the patient as well as for the doctor or nurse who performs it.

PRESSURE SORES

Pressure sores (decubitus ulcers, bedsores, ischaemic or trophic ulcers) are ulcerated areas of the skin occurring mainly over bony prominences of the skeleton and may be classified according to their size and depth of tissue destroyed. They have been the hallmark of the chronically ill, debilitated or disabled patient for centuries. They cause considerable distress to patients, delaying their recovery and causing much extra nursing. No precise figure for the incidence of new pressure sores is available but it has been estimated that there are at least 30 000 patients in the UK with pressure sores at any one time, such patients being nursed both at home in the community as well as in hospital.

Pressure sores should not be thought of as the responsibility only of the nursing staff. They are wounds of complex aetiology and pathology. Their prevention and treatment, as with many other areas of care of elderly patients, demands the expertise of a multidisciplinary team, including doctors.

Pathogenesis (Table 13.3)

The epidermis functions as a barrier between the tissues and organs of the body and the external environment. Like every other tissue, it requires an adequate blood supply bringing oxygen and nutrients and removing waste products to maintain its viability. Pressure and shear forces may interrupt the blood supply to the skin causing tissue ischaemia and, eventually, necrosis. However, the results of these forces will also depend on various intrinsic factors specific to each individual patient.

Table 13.3 *Development of pressure sores*

Primary factors
Pressure*—magnitude and duration
Shearing forces and friction
Predisposing factors
Immobility
Incontinence
Infection
Nutritional status
Anaemia and vascular disease
Neurological disease
Drugs

$$* \text{Pressure} = \frac{\text{Force}}{\text{Area}}$$

Pressure

Pressure on the surface of the skin will distort the underlying tissues. Pressure is the force exerted (in a perpendicular direction) over a given area, divided by that area. Therefore a large force may be dissipated over a large area, producing a very small pressure. Alternatively, a large force confined to a small area will generate a large pressure effect. The duration of pressure is as important as its magnitude, short periods of high pressure being as potentially damaging as prolonged periods of lower pressures. The dermis of the skin is often able to dissipate pressure effects. However, over bony prominences, it is relatively thin and therefore pressure here may distort blood vessels sufficiently to interrupt the blood supply. If this pressure persists for any length of time, cell death and tissue necrosis develop and a pressure sore will have begun. The majority of pressure sores occur below the waistline, common sites being over the sacrum, buttocks and heels.

Shearing forces

When pressure is applied at an angle to the skin surface, shearing forces are created as the various layers of the skin move over each other, causing tissue distortion. This may occur as friction between the skin and, for example, bed sheets during a poorly executed lift of a patient in bed. In an emaciated patient with lax skin, folding of the skin occurs with movement, causing further damage. Dermal capillaries may thus be stretched and compressed causing tissue ischaemia. As with pressure, the duration of the shear force is as important as its magnitude.

Intrinsic predisposing factors

There are also many intrinsic predisposing factors in the development of pressure sores, which are specific to the individual patient. Fit, healthy people constantly redistribute pressure on load-bearing areas by frequent conscious and subconscious movement, regardless of being awake or asleep. Reduced frequency of movement, caused by limited mobility and impaired sensation to pressure or pain, are high risk factor in the development of pressure sores and may occur in patients who have suffered strokes or who have spinal cord disease, multiple sclerosis or diabetes. Incontinence increases the risk of pressure sore development. By causing skin maceration and excoriation, the risk of friction is increased, as is the risk of superficial infection.

In general, thin people will have a thin dermis and less fat and muscle to dissipate applied pressure and will be at greater risk of developing pressure sores than those with more adipose tissue. However, although obese patients may be better 'cushioned' from direct pressure effects, they may be at greater risk of shearing forces due to handling difficulties by nursing staff.

A poor nutritional state or subclinical malnutrition prevents efficient cellular repair. Protein deficiency and deficiencies of vitamin C, D and zinc are associated with poor collagen formation, while anaemia increases the likelihood of pressure injury. Pyrexia associated with infection increases the metabolic rate, so increasing the demand for oxygen; hence the presence of infection may endanger existing ischaemic areas. Generalized diseases affecting tissue perfusion e.g. cardiac failure, diabetes, pulmonary disease producing hypoxia, also increase the likelihood of a patient developing a pressure sore. Drugs may also be implicated in their formation: sedatives reduce spontaneous movement, while the catabolic activity of corticosteroids and cytotoxic agents impedes tissue repair. It is therefore not surprising that elderly people, with their accumulation of degenerative diseases as well as the age-related thinning of their skin, are such good candidates for developing these sores when they become ill and less mobile.

Treatment (Table 13.4)

The treatment of pressure sores revolves around the relief of pressure to the skin and the removal or avoidance of any of the predisposing factors that had operated to increase the patient's vulnerability to their development.

Table 13.4 *Guidelines in treatment of pressure sores*

- Specific measures
  - Debride necrotic tissue
    - —surgical
    - —enzymatic
    - —chemical
  - Keep wound moist
  - Eradicate/prevent infection
- General measures
  - Relief of pressure and promotion of good skin care
  - Attention to general health of patient
    - —nutritional status
    - —cardiovascular and respiratory status
  - Promote mobility and continence
    (or lessen effects of incontinence)

As with any wound, healing of a pressure sore occurs by granulation and epithelialization if both the broken area and the surrounding tissue are healthy and moist and have an adequate blood supply. Healing of pressure sores may be slow in the presence of peripheral vascular disease or may not be achieved at all. Necrotic tissue prevents healing and must therefore be removed to produce a healthy granulation bed. Local debridement, with either a scalpel or by enzymatic or chemical means, may be used as part of the wound dressing. The presence of infection also delays healing and must be eradicated, but some bacteria will always be present in an open wound and therefore striving for sterility is unrealistic. Topical cleansing with normal saline solution is usually adequate and will not damage healthy tissue; systemic antibiotics should be reserved for infection with surrounding cellulitis. There is no place for topical antibiotics. Various functionally specific wound dressings are available to prevent dehydration and contamination, but the wounds must be assessed and the appropriate dressing applied correctly.

Repositioning schedules are vital for patients who are chair-bound or confined to bed, to prevent long periods of localized pressure. This may take the form of altering the patient's position every two hours, or as frequently as necessary for each patient. Various mechanical devices that alternate or redistribute pressure, or turn and tilt the patient at regular intervals, may assist in this purpose. If patients with impaired mobility are nursed in bed, bed cradles will support the bed linen away from the feet, while sheepskin boots will provide protection and comfort for the heels. It is important to beware the tendency of patients nursed in a semi-recumbent position in bed to slide down the bed. Wet bed linen or clothing from incontinence prevent good skin care and promote friction stresses on the skin as patients move. Promotion of continence is therefore of great importance but if this is not possible, a permanent indwelling catheter may be needed to protect the skin.

For patients with pressure sores as a whole, it is essential to optimize their general physical state as far as possible. In particular, cardiac failure or dependent oedema should be controlled, while respiratory function, if impaired, should be treated actively. A blood transfusion for moderately severe anaemia will accelerate healing and may be indicated in certain patients. Evidence of poor nutrition should be corrected and all patients should have a well-balanced diet. Patients should be encouraged to be as mobile as possible with the aid of the physiotherapist and occupational therapist.

Prevention

It is clear from the causative and predisposing factors that some patients are more likely to develop pressure sores than others. Their prevention centres around improving the mobility, continence and general health of patients, thereby making sure that pressure and shear forces on vulnerable areas of their skin are kept to a minimum. Many sophisticated techniques, such as thermography, are being developed to assess skin areas at risk, so that damaged areas are detected before there is any observable change on the skin surface.

Various clinically orientated rating scales that assess risk of developing pressure sores have been used as guides to enable rational prophylactic regimens to be used. The Norton Scale, for example, provides a scoring system for five important variables (Table 13.5). The lower the score, the greater the risk of developing pressure sores and therefore preventative measures must be taken. Patients must be assessed and reassessed regularly as their general condition changes. If these factors in the treatment of elderly patients are considered by all members of the multidisciplinary team, the incidence of pressure sores, with their attendant morbidity and mortality, will be reduced.

Table 13.5 *The Norton Scale: an assessment of risk of developing pressure sores (after Norton* et al. *1962)*

Score	*Physical condition*	*Mental state*	*Activity*	*Mobility*	*Incontinence*
4	Good	Alert	Ambulant	Full	Not
3	Fair	Apathetic	Walks/help	Slightly limited	Occasionally
2	Poor	Confused	Chairbound	Very limited	Usually/urine
1	Very bad	Stuporose	Bedfast	Immobile	Doubly

For each patient, score 1–4 under each heading and total the scores: patients with a total score of 14 or less are 'at risk'; 12 or less are 'at *high* risk' and preventative care is essential

Chapter

14

Terminal Care

PAIN • ANALGESIC AGENTS • OTHER SYMPTOMS OF THE TERMINALLY ILL • PSYCHOLOGICAL ASPECTS OF DYING • SPECIAL PROBLEMS IN ELDERLY PATIENTS

Effective management of terminally ill patients should be an important part of every doctor's basic knowledge. Whatever medical advances are made, no one lives for ever. Doctors must use their diagnostic skills and the drugs available to make all patients as comfortable as possible when they come to the end of their lives. The instinctive horror often accompanying the word 'cancer' is inexorably linked in the minds of many people with constant, uncontrolled pain. With current knowledge, such a situation should never happen.

The original concept of terminal care arose in patients suffering from cancer at a stage when active, curative treatment was no longer appropriate. It is often difficult for those attending such patients to switch from this 'curing' mode to one of 'caring', where assessment and investigations are directed towards controlling symptoms of an uncontrollable cancer rather than eradicating it. Such patients are often young. However, some elderly patients equally need the skills of good symptom control for their cancers.

This approach is also applicable to other elderly patients dying because of, for example, pneumonia secondary to cardiac failure, stroke, etc. Though chest infections are potentially curable with antibiotics and chest physiotherapy, there also may come a time when such therapy is inappropriate to a dying patient and a 'care mode' needed instead. The psychological needs of dying patients also have to be identified and, if possible, met. This may often be very difficult for the attending staff, who thereby have to face their own mortality, but it can be as rewarding as treating physical symptoms.

PAIN

Pain is not a simple sensation but a complex physical and emotional experience. Chronic pain is often difficult to describe or locate and may be seen by patients as an unending, meaningless endurance and an agonizing disintegration of their lives. To control pain effectively, the following steps are necessary:

1. Assess the severity of the pain.
2. Assess the cause of pain in order to give the most effective form of analgesia.
3. Use regular analgesia—in adequate doses to *prevent* pain recurring.
4. Give sympathy and understanding (antidepressants to elevate mood may occasionally be considered in addition).
5. Reassess regularly.

Severity of pain

A careful history of the pain is essential—its character (burning, stabbing, dull ache, etc.) and the factors altering its intensity. Is the pain less at rest than on movement, lying or standing? What makes it worse? Does anything relieve it—drugs, alcohol, heat from a hot water bottle, etc.? Is sleep disturbed or activity limited? A drug history is also essential—which drugs have failed, which have helped? Patients and their relatives (if at home) or the nurses (if in hospital) all need to be asked for this information, rather than waiting until the patients complain or admit to pain themselves.

Causes of pain (Table 14.1)

Tumour infiltration of bone

Infiltration of bone either by primary or metastatic tumour is the commonest cause of pain in advanced cancer. The characteristics of this type of pain vary with the site but it is generally constant and becomes progressively more severe. Many bony metastases produce a prostaglandin-like material, thought to be responsible for causing pain. Non-steroidal anti-inflammatory agents, which are potent inhibitors of prostaglandin synthesis, have been found particularly effective in relieving such bone pain.

Tumour infiltration of a nerve, plexus or root

Infiltration of neural structures causes constant burning pain, hyperaesthesia and paraesthesia followed by sensory loss. Pain from local bony involvement causing nerve root compression (as with a collapsed vertebra) may cause either local pain or radicular pain in the area served by the involved nerve. Symptoms vary according to the exact site of involvement and commonly include motor weakness, progressing to paralysis and altered sensation (i.e. hyperaesthesia or paraesthesia) that may be subjectively unpleasant, before progressing to sensory loss. If the autonomic nervous system is affected, bladder and bowel function will be impaired. Adrenal corticosteroids may cause a transient improvement in symptoms by reducing perineural oedema, but nerve blocks (e.g. using phenol), where possible, are the only means of abolishing such pain.

Tumour infiltration of viscera

Infiltration of visceral structures such as the biliary tract, stomach, ureters, uterus or bladder produces local tissue ischaemia that may be responsible for visceral pain, which is characteristically constant, diffuse and progressively increases in intensity. Such pain is best treated by a nerve block to the coeliac plexus or opiate analgesics.

Pleural pain

Tumour infiltration of the pleura causes pleuritic pain, worse on inspiration or coughing. Such pain is effectively treated by intercostal nerve blocks to the appropriate area.

Ascites

Tumour seedlings (e.g. from ovarian carcinoma) spread within the peritoneal endothelium from abdominal or pelvic organs and may secrete large volumes of protein-rich fluid, causing abdominal distension and discomfort. Drainage of such ascitic fluid by paracentesis may provide temporary relief, while a more permanent shunt of the fluid

Table 14.1 *Causes of pain*

Tumour infiltration of
—bone
—nerve, plexus or root
—visceral organs
—pleura
Pressure effects
—ascites
—lymphoedema
—cerebral tumour
Infection
Gastrointestinal obstruction
—tumour
—constipation
Immobility

into the thoracic duct or central venous system may need to be considered if rapid re-accumulation occurs. Instillation of cytotoxic agents into the peritoneal cavity is not generally effective.

Lymphoedema

Lymph accumulation in a limb occurs when tumour tissue obstructs the return of lymph from the limb, usually by infiltration of the draining lymph nodes. Tissue distension may cause discomfort, while the limb itself may be difficult to move because of its increased weight. Simple analgesia may have a place in the management of this condition, but mechanical intermittent compression of the arm or leg often reduces the swelling and hence relieves the discomfort considerably.

Headache

Headache may arise from raised intracranial pressure from a cerebral primary or metastatic tumour. High-dose corticosteroids may cause dramatic relief of pain by reducing cerebral oedema. Initially, dexamethasone (4 mg q.d.s. as a maximum dose) should be used, and if effective, reduced subsequently to the minimum level maintaining the improvement. When steroids are no longer effective, and if pain remains a major symptom, opiate analgesia is necessary.

Secondary infection

The secondary infection of a malignant ulcer or pressure sore may cause pain. It may be superficial, simply requiring regular cleansing with antiseptic solutions, or deep, when systemic antibiotic therapy is required.

Abdominal colic

Colic may be caused by intestinal obstruction due to tumour or to relative obstruction from hard intraluminal faeces i.e. constipation. The latter is eminently treatable by softening and bulk-forming agents and aperients, with the possible addition of an initial bowel movement derived from rectal enemas. Pain from impending intestinal obstruction caused by a primary or metastatic tumour may be relieved by softening agents and a semifluid diet (if the obstruction is not complete) or by the combination of analgesia and antispasmodic agents (e.g. hyoscine, which may be given parenterally).

Immobility

When a patient is dying, body movement is usually reduced so the risk of developing painful pressure sores is very high (*see* Chapter 13). Pain in a paralysed limb may be found in patients with carcinomatosis and paralysis secondary to nerve involvement. When such patients are terminally ill, nerve blocks should be considered, otherwise opiates remain the mainstay of treatment. However, patients who have suffered a stroke may also have painful dysaesthesia of their affected limbs, in addition to pain from hypertonicity. Hypertonic limbs may respond to antispasticity agents, but all causes of pain in a paralysed limb will gain benefit from physiotherapy and frequent passive movements.

Fear and anxiety

Finally, it must be remembered that the physical pain of a patient with a terminal illness is magnified subjectively by fear and anxiety—fear of the pain recurring, fear of death and anxiety about present and future interpersonal relationships, to name but a few. Such fears and anxieties must also be addressed and, hopefully, lessened for optimal pain control.

ANALGESIC AGENTS

The aim of analgesia should be to render the patient *pain free* at all times. As mentioned earlier, corticosteroids and non-steroidal anti-inflammatory drugs may be very effective agents in controlling certain types of pain. The severity of pain will indicate whether mild analgesics are required or whether stronger opiate analgesics are necessary. A patient may only require mild analgesia for most of the time, but for intermittent painful procedures, such as dressing changes, nitrous oxide and oxygen in equal parts (Entonox), or sublingual buprenorphine (Temgesic), will often provide temporary, heightened analgesia. Mild analgesic agents include soluble aspirin and paracetamol, which can be given four to six hourly. If these are ineffective, weak opiates (dihydrocodeine (DF118), codeine phosphate or dextropropoxyphene combined with paracetamol (Co-codamol or Coproxamol)) may be tried instead.

More severe pain will require the stronger opiates for adequate control. In this category, diamorphine or morphine are the drugs of choice (10 mg oral diamorphine is equivalent to 15 mg oral morphine). They are extremely potent and versatile analgesics, offering several routes of administration in addition to various oral presentations (Table 14.2). The major advantage of diamorphine over morphine is its higher water solubility so that different strength oral solutions can easily be made. Diamorphine is rapidly metabolized in the body and probably exerts its effects through several metabolites, one of which is morphine. However, diamorphine in solution is unstable, with a shelf life of only three to four weeks. As diamorphine and morphine have a duration of action of approximately four hours, doses therefore must be repeated every four hours. A patient's pain should be titrated against increasing doses of four-hourly diamorphine, until control is achieved. At this point, the analgesia may be changed to a more convenient form, i.e. twice daily controlled release tablets or a continuous subcutaneous infusion.

Psychological dependence is not observed in terminally ill patients. Similarly, tolerance to analgesia does not occur, though tolerance to side-effects such as drowsiness and nausea develops after a few days.

Table 14.2 *Strong opiate analgesics*

Drug	*Route of admission*	*Dose interval*	*Comments*
Diamorphine elixir	Oral*	Every 4 hours	Useful to titrate pain to bring it under control initially
Diamorphine	Subcutaneous or Intramuscular	Every 4 hours	Useful for patients unable to swallow
Diamorphine	Subcutaneous	Continuous infusion via infusion pump	Offers convenience especially if patient at home; infusion pump may be primed by District Nurse every 24 hours
Morphine	Per rectum	Every 4 hours	Useful for selected patients to avoid oral and subcutaneous routes
Diamorphine	Intravenous	Every 4 hours	Repeated doses to be avoided; they result in higher peak levels which will produce more side-effects and give no better control than regular s.c. injections
Morphine sulphate in controlled release tablets	Oral	Every 12 hours	Convenient and effective twice daily dosage; formulation of the tablets makes 24-hour total dose of diamorphine equipotent with controlled release morphine
Buprenorphine (Temgesic)	Sublingual	Every 6–8 hours	Has ceiling effect of analgesia; partial agonist activity, therefore will reduce concurrent opiate therapy

* Diamorphine: 20 mg oral is equivalent to 10 mg by subcutaneous route

Opiate requirements may, however, rise over a period of time, but this usually reflects increasing pain from progressive disease. Regular prophylactic laxatives must always be prescribed when opiates are used, as constipation invariably occurs.

OTHER SYMPTOMS OF THE TERMINALLY ILL (Table 14.3)

Respiratory symptoms

Dyspnoea

Either at rest or on minimal exertion, dyspnoea may be a presenting symptom in the presence of a pulmonary carcinoma, metastatic effusion or infection. It may also be caused by bronchospasm or pulmonary oedema, both eminently treatable. If a malignant pleural effusion is causing distress, temporary benefit may be given by draining it to dryness and instilling a fibrotic agent, e.g. tetracycline, to prevent or delay the re-accumulation of fluid. Dyspnoea may also result from restricted movement of the lungs because of the presence of large volumes of ascitic fluid. In such cases treatment of the ascites will relieve the dyspnoea (*see* p. 156). The sensation of dyspnoea secondary to intrapulmonary metastases or lymphangitis carcinomatosis may be alleviated by dexamethasone, but small doses of diamorphine are often needed in addition.

Cough and excessive bronchial secretions

Both cough and copious bronchial secretions may cause distress in dying patients with malignancy and those with non-malignant terminal illness. A troublesome cough may be alleviated by linctus with sedative properties, e.g. codeine linctus. Bronchial secretions may be reduced by atropine-like agents, e.g. hyoscine.

The question of whether or not to treat a chest infection with antibiotics in a patient with a terminal illness is difficult to answer in general terms. Good symptom control must always be paramount, e.g. controlling pleuritic pain, a productive cough, etc. The correct and most appropriate mode of treatment must be decided with each individual patient.

Table 14.3 *Common symptoms of terminally ill patients*

Pain
Respiratory
—dyspnoea
—cough and excessive bronchial secretions
Central nervous system
—headache
—agitation and restlessness
—anxiety and depression
—insomnia
Gastrointestinal
—anorexia
—nausea and vomiting
—constipation
—intestinal obstruction
—mouth problems
Skin
—ulcers
—odours
—pruritus
Incontinence

Central nervous system symptoms

Headache

Headache arising from intracerebral tumours may respond to high dose corticosteroids (*see* p. 157). If there are accompanying focal neurological signs, these may sometimes improve with palliative whole-brain irradiation, with coincident improvement in the quality of life (at the expense of alopecia).

Agitation and restlessness

Agitation may arise from anxiety, or be the result of pain, constipation, or urinary retention. The last three physical conditions are readily treatable. However, drug therapy may be necessary for agitated patients who are mentally confused and for whom there is no apparent physical reason for their agitation. For such patients, one of the phenothiazine drugs e.g. thioridazine should be used, starting with a small dose and increasing as necessary.

If patients are so confused and agitated that they continually refuse all oral medication, fluphenazine, as a single depot intramuscular injection, may have a sustained calming effect. The response to 12.5 mg fluphenazine should be observed initially and increased or repeated at 2–4 week intervals, as needed.

Anxiety and depression

Symptoms of anxiety and depression are often considered 'natural' in a patient who is terminally ill. Natural apprehension about the future course of the illness needs to be distinguished from anxiety; sadness from true depression. Both may respond to sympathetic counselling and support by those caring for them. Drug therapy is a poor substitute for this personal involvement, but may be justified in particularly distressed patients, in addition to such counselling.

Insomnia

Lack of sleep may reflect physical symptoms, such as pain, and psychological problems, such as anxiety and depression. Such problems need to be addressed directly, but hypnotics may also be necessary.

Gastrointestinal symptoms

Anorexia

Anorexia may have many causes, e.g. uncontrolled pain, sore mouth, nausea, constipation. Alternatively, it may be a feature of the terminal illness itself and not require treatment.

Nausea and vomiting

These also have many causes. The vomiting centre in the medulla can be stimulated in several ways:

1. Via higher centres, e.g. anxiety.
2. Directly, e.g. opiates, radiotherapy, raised intracranial pressure.
3. Via the chemoreceptor trigger zone, e.g. opiates, hypercalcaemia, uraemia.
4. Via vagal and sympathetic afferent fibres, e.g. from the pharynx

(cough); gut irritation—pressure (from intestinal obstruction or constipation); or chemical (e.g. drugs).

Specific causes must always be treated first, such as clearing constipation, though non-specific anti-emetic drugs may also need to be used. The choice of an anti-emetic depends on its site of action and possible side-effects, also its availability as a suppository, thus avoiding the need for injections.

Constipation

Constipation must be considered in every patient and prevented, if possible. Treatment is obligatory in patients receiving opiates. The small quantities of food, low in fibre, and insufficient fluid intake of many patients with terminal illnesses, in addition to the various drugs they are prescribed, conspire to cause intestinal stasis. Drugs that act as faecal softeners, osmotic agents and colonic stimulants are helpful taken orally, as prophylaxis. Hard, impacted faeces in the rectum will need local treatment with suppositories, enemas or occasionally, manual evacuation.

Intestinal obstruction

Obstruction due to malignancy may cause nausea, vomiting and abdominal colic. Pain may be relieved by analgesics and antispasmodic agents; nausea by anti-emetics, given rectally or by injection. However, such measures are liable, together with the patient's small food and liquid intake, to increase the risk of incomplete obstruction becoming complete by causing constipation as well. Hence a stool softener without stimulant activity is essential. If the site of the obstruction is distal to the duodenum, there is usually absorption of sufficient fluid to prevent severe dehydration. Symptoms of thirst are rare, whereas complaints of a dry mouth are common and should always be alleviated. Nasogastric intubation and intravenous hydration are seldom needed in the last days or weeks of life.

Mouth problems

Oral problems are extremely common and easily overlooked. Good oral hygiene prevents soreness and infection of the mouth and gums. A dry mouth may result from dehydration or be a side-effect of drugs with anticholinergic properties, e.g. phenothiazines and tricyclic antidepressants. Simple local measures, such as giving crushed ice or frozen tonic water to suck, are often successful. Monilial (Candida) infection may cause a red sore mouth in addition to the more easily recognized white plaques. Oesophageal involvement by monilial infection will cause painful dysphagia. Antifungal agents, e.g. nystatin in the form of lozenges or a suspension, will rapidly eradicate this infection.

Hypercalcaemia

Hypercalcaemia is a frequent consequence of disseminated malignancy, especially from carcinoma of the breast, prostate and thyroid, and from myelomatosis. Typical symptoms are thirst, anorexia, nausea, vomiting and constipation—all of which are common in patients who are terminally ill anyway. Treatment of mild or moderate hypercalcaemia, when responsible for such symptoms, is worthwhile because the quality of life is often substantially improved. Initial treatment is directed towards correcting dehydration, which is always associated with it, by oral or intravenous rehydration, combined with frusemide to promote calcium excretion. Oral or intravenous phosphate may be added, while the effect of high-dose corticosteroids may be effective in lowering the serum calcium after a two to three day delay. Other drugs used to lower hypercalcaemia, e.g. salmon calcitonin and mithramycin, are inappropriate for the terminally ill.

Dermatological problems

Ulcers

Ulcers over pressure areas may be painful or cause an offensive odour. Their treatment is considered in Chapter 13. Malignant ulcers may be similarly treated by debridement of slough and cleansing with antiseptic solutions. Palliative radiotherapy should be considered for all fungating tumours.

Odours

These are usually the result of infection, which must therefore be treated by local methods (*see* above). Foul-smelling odours are associated with the presence of anaerobic bacteria, for which metronidazole is the antibiotic of choice (given orally or by suppository). If these methods are not successful or there is a colostomy or permanent discharge present, adsorbents such as charcoal dressings may be useful to isolate and contain the odour.

Pruritus

Itching, when a result of jaundice and increased bile salts in the blood, may be helped by the chelating agent, cholestyramine. Other causes of pruritus are poorly understood but non-specific measures, e.g. cooling with fans, emollient creams or the sedative effect of systemic antihistamines should always be tried if the symptom is troublesome.

Urinary incontinence

Urinary incontinence may be an extremely uncomfortable and unpleasant experience, especially for a dying patient. It may be precipitated by faecal impaction or the excessive diuresis caused by powerful diuretics, hyperglycaemia or hypercalcaemia, all of which are amenable to treatment. Inappropriate diuretic therapy should be withdrawn whenever possible. Male patients may also have the additional problem of prostatism, causing urinary retention with overflow. However, urinary incontinence may also be a feature of progressive mental impairment and uninhibited bladder activity. In all instances where continence cannot be regained, long-term bladder catheterization should be considered, both to prevent the discomfort of wet clothing and the surrounding skin from becoming macerated.

PSYCHOLOGICAL ASPECTS OF DYING

The process of dying of a terminally ill patient involves a metaphorical journey towards understanding and acceptance of this knowledge. It is often a slow process during which the patient's situation, insight and needs are constantly changing. The decision to tell patients that they have an incurable illness may be debated endlessly. However, a better question to ask is *how much* of the truth may be given at each particular stage of the illness. As with other aspects of geriatric care, it is helpful to see each patient in her social context, together with the spouse, close family or friends. An advantage of cancer as a potentially fatal illness is that it gives time—time to the patient, the family and carers to come to terms with the realities of the illness and for the changes which will come about when that patient dies.

As with other major life changes, there are two main components in the acceptance of a terminal illness. There is the initial fear and apprehension—of the process of dying, of loss of control, of the separation from family, home, etc. Discussion of these fears needs to be encouraged with effective communication between the patient and the carers. Then follows a period of grieving: at first, incomprehension and numbness may be followed by a period of intense inner struggling to retain the status quo, leading to a phase of dejection and hopelessness. Finally, little by little, acceptance of the 'new order' is achieved to replace the old. Older people generally accept the possibility of their dying more easily than younger people, with the result that its acceptance may be reached relatively quickly. However, understanding the problems facing each patient is necessary, as some, like their younger counterparts, pass painfully through each phase in their psychological journey.

Bereavement

Those who have been bereaved face similar transition periods to those of the dying patient in their grief reaction before achieving the final realization and acceptance of their situation. Time before the anticipated death of a spouse or loved one may have given the opportunity to resolve differences and develop the relationship that existed. However, subsequently, there is the need to express grief. Such expressed grief is frequently shunned and causes embarrassment in our society, which as a whole has great difficulty in coming to terms with death. Bereavement remains one of the commonest causes of suicide; if the bereaved person is isolated from family and friends, the dangers of suicide must be carefully assessed. In the first year after bereavement, the incidence of disease, morbidity and death itself are also increased in those close relatives who are left. Symptoms must therefore always be considered carefully in patients who have recently been bereaved and not automatically ascribed simply to sadness or depression.

SPECIAL PROBLEMS IN ELDERLY PATIENTS

The Hospice Movement has brought about greater awareness and improved care of patients dying from cancer. In the elderly population, death is less likely to result from malignant disease than from cardiovascular and cerebrovascular causes. About a third of patients admitted to acute geriatric units die there, usually from ostensibly treatable conditions like cardiac failure or chest infections. Here the diagnosis of dying is often made by exclusion, by the failure of response to standard therapeutic and rehabilitative endeavours. Also, the duration of the terminal illness may be quite short, with little time to readjust patient care from a 'cure mode' to a 'care mode', and thus provide good symptom control and psychological support.

Terminal care of elderly patients may be further compounded by difficulties in communication. Deafness and failing eyesight are readily understood, with some means available to overcome them. However, dying patients may be acutely confused, e.g. due to hypoxia from cardiac failure, or chronically confused from a dementing illness, such that speech may be extremely limited or inappropriate. Confusion and distress may, however, occur together. Attempts must always be made to alleviate the distress, mental or physical, by careful observation of non-verbal information together with an understanding of likely problems.

In an ideal world, the dying patient is seen as part of a close social network, with family and friends providing additional comfort and support. Such people themselves are a source of much useful background information about the patient, which is of considerable help to the attending hospital staff. Elderly people admitted to hospital are more likely to be socially isolated than their younger counterparts. It is not unknown for dying elderly patients to have no family or friends visit them while in hospital. This places increased demands on the nursing staff, which are not readily met on a busy hospital ward. However, in some hospitals, volunteer visitors are increasingly being used in this important role.

With the expected dramatic rise in the number of elderly people over the next 20 years, the number of such patients ending their lives in hospital will also rise substantially. Their special needs must be recognized before they can be provided with the terminal care appropriate for them.

Appendix

1

Areas for Future Research

Although Geriatric Medicine is a comparatively new medical speciality, it encompasses medical problems that have been known for many years. Fields of fruitful research are numerous and can be found in every aspect of the speciality. They can be divided roughly into three broad areas: (i) basic scientific research; (ii) study of disease processes; and (iii) epidemiological and sociological aspects of ageing and disease.

Gerontology, the study of ageing, is a rapidly expanding field of specific research. The regulation of growth and differentiation and the mechanisms underlying unregulated growth, i.e. neoplasia, have attracted the attention of scientists for many years, but there is now considerable interest in uncovering the mechanisms that govern a cell's (or organism's) natural life-span, and the processes underlying 'natural' degeneration, as distinct from those superimposed by disease. Knowledge about 'normal' structure and function in man has generally been confined to that occurring in *young* adults, but much more awareness (and knowledge) is needed of 'normal' ageing processes.

The nature of various diseases has long been studied so that better means of amelioration or cure may become available. The scientific basis for understanding many of the degenerative diseases, such as osteoarthritis, dementia or vascular disease, covers areas that have excited the interest of doctors from many different specialities for many years. Treatment of such diseases remains rudimentary and more research is urgently needed so that some impact can be made in reducing the toll of suffering they produce.

For pharmacologists, the differences and similarities of drug handling and their effects in elderly people, compared with younger adults, is an important area of research which has only recently become widely recognized. As elderly people are the target for a high proportion of the nation's drug prescribing, such research has immense practical and economic implications.

Until recently, there were few hard facts about the size of the many common medical problems that afflict elderly people. Some questions of this nature, which have only been looked at in the last 20 years include: how common are falls among elderly people, and what are they caused by?—what is the prevalence of dementia and other organic brain pathology in the community?—and how common is hospital admission related to the administration of drugs? Answers to these and other similar questions are of great practical importance in the planning of health care in the community, as well as directing the attention of doctors who work in hospitals to common medical problems affecting elderly people in our society.

The cumulative effects of ageing and disease and the changing population structure of our society which bears them are relatively new phenomena. The structure of society in the year 2000 will be vastly different from what it was in 1900, and yet there is little awareness of what practical social, political and economic changes are going to be necessary to accommodate this. These changes will occur in the lifetime of most of the readers of this short book; they offer us the challenge of improving the medical care of elderly people and, thereby, the quality of life for future generations.

Appendix

2

Training and Career Opportunities

It was not long ago that Geriatric Medicine was notable by its absence from the medical curriculum of the majority of medical schools in the UK. Over the past 10 years, this situation has changed so that most medical students now, to a greater or lesser extent, have some undergraduate experience of the speciality. The rapid growth in the numbers of elderly people has created the need for expert medical care which is specifically geared to them. There are now 23 University Departments of Geriatric Medicine in the UK and many new consultant posts have been created throughout the country (sometimes from existing general medical posts), which thereby recognize the demands of the changing age structure of our population. Geriatric Medicine forms the third largest speciality within medicine and has over 500 consultant posts in the country.

The training requirements for a career in hospital-orientated Geriatric Medicine are similar to those for any other medical speciality in the UK, i.e. there must be a sound grounding in General Medicine and the attainment of Membership of the Royal College of Physicians (MRCP) before specialist training in Geriatric Medicine is begun. Posts at Senior House Officer (SHO) or Registrar level in almost any medical speciality will be useful in the future (but especially Neurology, Rheumatology, Gastroenterology, Cardiology and Respiratory Medicine). Indeed, geriatricians of today have brought past experience from many different specialities to their present work with elderly patients. Many medical rotations include posts in Geriatric Medicine, which give young doctors some experience in the speciality and a chance to discover whether they find the work satisfying.

Some doctors who are particularly interested in an academic career enter a research post at this stage, while others undertake research projects as Senior Registrars. Such research may lead to a higher qualification, such as an MD or PhD. A Senior Registrar appointment is necessary for higher specialist training in Geriatric Medicine and is usually for four years. Such posts provide specific experience in most aspects of care of elderly patients: work on acute and rehabilitation wards, long-stay wards, day hospital and outpatient work, domiciliary visiting and liaison with doctors in other specialities, paramedical staff and community workers. Training may be in Geriatric Medicine alone, or Geriatric Medicine combined with General Medicine, for those who wish to pursue a career as a General Physician with special responsibility for the elderly. Competition for Consultant posts is becoming more intense, but there is a continual small number of posts becoming vacant, Geriatric Medicine being one of the few expanding medical specialities at the present time.

GERIATRIC MEDICINE AND GENERAL PRACTICE

Elderly people form a substantial part of the workload of most general practitioners. In recognition of the importance of understanding how to treat elderly people, SHO posts in Geriatric Medicine are frequently included in General Practice vocational training schemes. The Royal College of Physicians has recently introduced an examination for the Diploma in Geriatric Medicine (DGM), which is designed for general practitioners who wish to extend and deepen their knowledge of the overall management of elderly patients. It takes the form of a written paper of short questions followed by a clinical examination. Further details about the examination and its syllabus can be obtained from the Royal College of Physicians, 11 St Andrews Place, Regents Park, London NW1 4LE.

Appendix

3

References and Further Reading

COMPREHENSIVE REFERENCE BOOKS

Brocklehurst J. C., ed. (1985). *Textbook of Geriatric Medicine and Gerontology* 3rd edn. Edinburgh: Churchill Livingstone.

Pathy M. S. J., ed. (1985). *Principles and Practice of Geriatric Medicine*. Chichester: John Wiley and Sons.

BOOKS ON VARIOUS ASPECTS OF GERIATRIC MEDICINE

Age Concern (1986). *The Law and Vulnerable Elderly People*. London: Age Concern.

Arie T., ed. (1985). *Recent Advances in Psychogeriatrics*. Edinburgh: Churchill Livingstone.

Brocklehurst J. C., ed. (1984). *Urology in the Elderly*. Edinburgh: Churchill Livingstone.

Goodwill C. J., Chamberlain M. A., eds. (1988). *Rehabilitation of the Physically Disabled Patient*. London: Croom Helm.

Hellemans J., Vantrappen G., eds. (1984). *Gastrointestinal Tract Disorders in the Elderly*. Edinburgh: Churchill Livingstone.

Mulley G. P. (1985). *Practical Management of Stroke*. London: Croom Helm.

Redfern S. J., ed. (1986). *Nursing Elderly People*. Edinburgh: Churchill Livingstone.

Saunders C. M., ed. (1978). *The Management of Terminal Disease*. London: Edward Arnold.

Swift C. G., ed. (1987). *Clinical Pharmacology in the Elderly*. New York: Marcel Dekker Inc.

Tallis R., ed. (1989). *The Clinical Neurology of Old Age*. Chichester: John Wiley and Sons.
Wells N., Freer C., eds. (1988). *The Ageing Population: Burden or Challenge*. London: Macmillan Press.

SPECIALIST JOURNALS

Age and Ageing (The official journal of the British Geriatrics Society and of the British Society for Research on Ageing).
Gerontology—International Journal of Experimental and Clinical Gerontology.
Journal of the American Geriatrics Society.
Also various articles on Geriatric Medical topics in general journals, e.g. *Lancet*, *British Medical Journal*, *British Journal of Hospital Medicine*.

SERIES OF BOOKS

Caird F. I., Grimley Evans J., eds. *Advanced Geriatric Medicine* (a series of books). London: Pitman Books.
Isaacs B., ed. *Recent Advances in Geriatric Medicine* (a series of books). Edinburgh: Churchill Livingstone.

Index

Abdominal colic 158
α-adrenergic blocking drugs 36, 142
Acetazolamide 91
Ageing 8–15
  biological process 7
  effect on organ systems 9–10
  precocious 14–15
  theories 10–13
    cellular mortality 11–12
    cross linkage 13
    immunological 12
    nucleic acid immobilization 13
    rate of living 12
    somatic mutation 12–13
    waste products 13
    wear and tear 12
Age-pigment (lipofuscin) 13, 14
Age-structure of society 1–2, 3 (table)
  men/women balance 2
Agnosia 53, 68–9
  spatial 68–9
  tactile (asterognosis) 68
  visual neglect 69
Albumin 29, 38, 39, 133
Alcoholism 45–7, 57, 102
Alzheimer's disease 51
Amantidine 79–80
Amaurosis fugax 73
Aminoglycosides 37, 95
Anaemia 39–42, 49, 95, 106, 122
  associated with malabsorption 43–5
  iron deficiency 41–2
  pernicious anaemia 40–1, 122
  preoperative 118
Analgesics 30, 159
  opiate analgesics 147, 159–61
Angiotensin-converting enzyme inhibitors 36
Antacids 36
Antibiotics 37
Anticholinergic drugs 79, 119, 139, 147
Anticonvulsants 30, 45
Antihypertensive therapy 36
Aphasia 53, 67
Apraxia 53, 69
Arthropathies 106, 115
Ascites 156–7
Ascorbic acid *see* Vitamin C
Aspirin 72, 159
Astereognosis (tactile agnosia) 68
Ataxia 68, 73
Atheroma 64
Attendance Allowance 25
Attitudes towards old age 7–8
Auditory system, age related changes 92–3
Autoimmune thyroiditis 121

Barbiturates 49, 55
β-blockers 29, 30, 95, 101, 125
Bedsores *see* Pressure sores
Benzerazide 79
Benzodiazepines 30, 55, 95, 101
Bereavement 49, 57, 167
Blindness, 69, 74, 87–8
  consequences 88
Blood pressure regulation 100
Bone, tumour infiltration of 155
Bouchard's nodes 110
Brain failure, chronic (long-standing confusion) 50
Bromocriptine 79
Buprenorphine (*Temgesic*) 159, 160 (table)
Burns 103
Butyrophenones 34, 101

Calciferol 47

Calcitonin 135
Calcium 42
  corrected calcium 133
Calcium antagonists 36
Calculi bladder 143, 144
Candidal (monilial) infection 165
Carbenoxolone 36
Carbidopa 79
Carbimazole 125
Cardiac dysrthythmias 49, 83, 95, 99
Carotid sinus hypersensitivity 102
Cartilage 109
Cataract 88–9
Cauda equina lesion 140, 145
Cellular mortality/immortality 11–12
Central retinal artery occlusion 90
Central retinal vein occlusion 90
Cerebellar ataxia 105
Cerebral circulation 63–4
Cervical spondylosis 85
Chlormethiazole 55
Chlorpromazine 55
Chlorpropamide 128
Chronic subdural haematoma 84
Cimetidine 36–7
Co-codamol 159
Codeine phosphate 159
Coeliac disease 43
Colchicine 45
Community psychogeriatric nurse 56
Community support 6–7
Compulsory care 60–2
Confusion 48–50
  acute 48–50
  persistent (chronic brain failure) 50
  postoperative 119
Constipation 81, 138, 147–8, 164
Continence 136–8
Coproxamol 159
Cortical blindness 69
Corticosteroids 114–15, 159, 162
Court of Protection 59
Crohn's disease 43, 44
Crush fractures 131, 134
Cystometry 143
Cystoscopy 144
Cysto-urethrography 143
Cytotoxic agents 43, 45

Day Centre 6, 26, 56
Day Hospital 26–7
Deafness 92–4
  management 93–4
Deep vein thrombosis 119
Dementia 45–6, 50–6, 57, 78, 105, 139
  Alzheimer's 15, 51
  diagnosis 52–4
    differential 53
  management 54–6
    disordered behaviour 54–5
    environment 55–6
    institutional care 56
  multi-infarct 51
  neurological diseases associated 51–2
Deprenyl 79
Depression 49, 57–8, 71, 78, 105, 147, 163
Detrusor instability ('unstable bladder') 138–9
Dexamethasone 157
DF118 (dihydrocodeine) 159
Diabetes mellitus 66, 81, 106, 126–9, 140, 141
  dietary advice 128
  insulin 128–9
  oral hypoglycaemic drugs 128
  retinopathy 91–2, 127
Diabetic ketoacidosis 49
Diamorphine 159, 160 (table); *see also* Opiate analgesics
Diarrhoea 146
  overflow 148
Dicopic test 41
Digoxin, 30, 34–5, 49, 95, 124
Dihydrocodeine (DF118) 159
Diogenes syndrome 58
Diphosphonates 135
Diploma in Geriatric Medicine 172
Disease presentation, altered 17
Diuretics 35–6, 95, 101, 147

urinary incontinence due to 142
Dizziness 95
Dopamine 77, 79
Dopamine-receptor blockers 34
Down's syndrome 15
Drop attacks 85, 99
Drugs 28–37
adverse reactions 28
associated with hypothermia 81–2
patient compliance 31
pharmacodynamics 30
pharmacokinetics 29–30
pre-operative 118
prescribing problems 31–2
record card (Camberwell) 33 (fig.)
Dysarthria 67

Effort syndrome 102
Entonox 159
Ephedrine 142
Epilepsy 66, 85, 99

Faecal impaction 138, 148, 164
Faecal incontinence 6, 145–7
laundry service 6
Falls 96–104
causes 98–103
external 98–9
iatrogenic 103
intrinsic 99–103
consequences 103–4
Family support 2–3
Faradism 138
Femoral neck fracture 116
Fibroblasts 11–12, 14
Fludrocortisone 101
Fluphenazine 162
Folic acid 40, 46
deficiency 40, 46

Gagenhalten (paratonic rigidity) 21
Gastric surgery 43, 44
Gentamycin 37
Giant cell arteritis (temporal arteritis) 74
Glaucoma
closed angle 91
open angle 89–90
Gliclazide 128
Gluten-sensitive enteropathy 44
Gold 115

Haloperidol 34, 55
Hashimoto's disease 122
Headache 157, 162
Hearing aids 93
Heberden's nodes 110
Hepatic microsomal enzymes 30
Hip replacement 116–17
History taking 17–19
Home help service 6, 25, 56
Homeostasis, age-related changes 30
Hospice movement 168
Huntington's disease (chorea) 51, 76
Hydrocephalus, normal pressure 84
Hydroxycobalamin 41
Hypercalcaemia 142, 147, 165
Hyperosmolar non-ketotic coma 129
Hypertension 64
Hyperthyroidism 49, 105, 123–5
causes 123–4
clinical features 124–5
diagnosis 125
treatment 125
Hypnotics 32–4
Hypocalcaemia 134
Hypoglycaemia 49, 66
Hypokalaemia 36, 49, 83, 102, 103, 106
Hypokinesia 77
Hypothermia 81–3, 103
causes 81–2
clinical features 82–3
prevention 83
treatment 83
Hypothyroidism (myxoedema) 49, 57, 82, 105, 121–3, 147
causes 121–2
clinical features 122–3
diagnosis 123
treatment 123

Iatrogenic disability disease 17, 102, 107
Immobility 104–7

Immobility – cont.
causes 105 (table), 105–7
drug therapy 107
local 105–6
psychological 106–7
systemic 106
Impaired autonomic function 80–1
Incontinence
faecal 145
urinary 136–45
Insulin 128–9
Intestinal ischaemia, chronic 44
Intestinal obstruction 164
Iodine 125
Iron deficiency 41–2
alcoholism associated 45
post-gastric surgery 43–4
Isolation 4–5, 57
Isoprenaline 30

Jakob–Creutzfeldt disease 51
Joint pain, causes of 115 (table)

Korsakoff's syndrome (psychosis) 45, 47
Kyphoscoliosis 22, 109
Kyphosis 132

Laxatives 147–8
L-dopa 101
Legal aspects of mental disorder 58–62
Lipofuscin (age-pigment) 13, 14
Living conditions 5–6
Longevity 13–14
Looser's zones (pseudo-fractures) 134
Lymphoedema 157

Madopar 79
Malabsorption syndromes 43–5
biliary disease associated 44
drugs associated 45
gastric surgery induced 43–4
pancreatic disease associated 44
small bowel pathology associated 44
systemic disease associated 45
Malnutrition 38
associated factors 46 (table)
high-risk groups 46–7
Married couples 5
'Meals on wheels' 6, 25, 47, 56
Menière's disease 95
Meningism 66–7
Menopause 2, 130
Mental Health Act 1983 61–2
Mental state 19–20
Mental status questionnaire 19, 20 (table), 52
Metabolic bone disease 129–35
Metformin 128
Methotrexate 45
Methyl dopa 36, 57
Micturition 136–7
syncope 102
Monilia (Candida) infection 165
Morphine 159, 160 (table); *see also* Opiate analgesics
Mouth problems 22–3, 164–5
Multidisciplinary rehabilitation team 23, 70
Multiple pathology 16–17
Muscular rigidity 77, 82
Myocardial infarct 17, 49, 100, 119
Myopathies 102
Myxoedema *see* Hypothyroidism

National Assistance Act 1948, Section 47 60–1
Neomycin 45
Nerves, tumour infiltration of 156
Nicotinic acid 46
Non-steroidal anti-inflammatory drugs 30, 37, 159
for:
osteoarthritis 111
rheumatoid arthritis 114–15
Normal pressure hydrocephalus 52, 84
Norton Scale 153 (fig.)
Nucleic acid immobilization 13
Nutrition 38–47
multiple deficiencies 43–5
Nystatin 165

Occupational therapy 24–5, 70
Oral hypoglycaemic drugs 128
Orthopaedic patient management 117–20
  postoperative complications 118–20
    cardiovascular 119
    confusion 119
    pressure sore 120
    respiratory 118–19
    stroke 119
  pre-operative assessment 117–18
  rehabilitation 120
Orthostatic hypotension *see* Postural hypotension
Osteitis deformans (Paget's disease) 134–5
Osteoarthritis 105, 108–12
  clinical features 109–10
  radiological features 113 (table)
  treatment 110–12
Osteoarthrosis, primary generalized 110
Osteomalacia 44, 45, 47, 102–3, 105, 132–4
  clinical features 133
  treatment 134
  X-ray changes 133–4
Osteoporosis (osteopenia) 105, 130–2
  clinical features 131
  prevention 132
  treatment 132
  types of 130
  X-ray changes 131
Otosclerosis 94–5
Overflow diarrhoea 148

Paget's disease (osteitis deformans) 105, 134–5
Pain 155–9
  causes 155–9
  severity 155
Paracetamol 159
Paraphrenia 58
Paratonic rigidity (*Gagenhalten*) 21
Parkinsonism 75–80, 99, 106, 139
  biochemistry 77
  clinical features 77–8
  histology 76–7
  treatment 78–80
    drug therapy 79
  types 75–6
d-penicillamine 115
Perforation of large bowel 17
Peripheral neuropathy 105
Pernicious anaemia 40–1, 122
Phenothiazines 34, 101
Phenytoin 37
Physical examination 19–23
  alimentary tract 22–3
  cardiovascular 22
  mental state 19–20
  neurological 21–2
  respiratory 22
Physiotherapy 23–4
  in Parkinson's disease 78
  after stroke 70
Pick's disease 51
Platelet aggregation 72
Pleural pain 156
Pneumonia 17
Polymyalgia rheumatica 74, 105
Postural hypotension (orthostatic hypotension) 22, 78, 80, 100–2, 105
  causes 101 (table)
  drug-induced 101 (table)
  management 101–2
Postural sway 96–7
Posture 78, 96–7
  sway 96–7
Power of Attorney 60
  enduring 60
Prazosin 36, 142
Prednisolone 74
Presbyacusis 10 (table), 94
Presbyopia 10, 86
Presentation of disease 17–19
Pressure sores 103, 105, 106, 120, 148–53, 165
  Norton Scale 153
  pathogenesis 149–51
    intrinsic predisposing factors 150–1
    pressure 149–50

Pressure sores – cont.
shearing forces 150
prevention 153
treatment 151–2
Probantheline 139
Prochlorperazine 34
Progeria 14
Propranolol 29, 30
Prostatic hypertrophy 23, 138, 144
Protein supplements 47
Pruritus 166
Pulmonary embolism 100, 119
Pyrexia 17
Pyridoxine 46

Rehabilitation team 120
Research areas 169–70
Residual urine 140, 143
Retinal detachment 91
Retirement 3–4
Rheumatoid arthritis 105, 112–15
clinical features 112
radiological features 113 (table)
treatment 113–15
drugs 114–15
surgery 115
Romberg test 97

Sacral bladder centre 137
Schilling test 41
Scurvy 39, 49
Section 47, National Assistance Act 1948 60–1
Sedatives 32–4, 54–5
Senile macular degeneration 88
Sensory inattention 68
Shy-Drager syndrome 80
Sinemet 79
Small bowel resection 44
Social work 23, 25–6
Speech therapist 23, 70
Steatorrhoea 44
Stress incontinence 138
Stroke 63–72, 105
causes 64–5
clinical features 67–9
apraxia 69
balance 68
communication difficulties 67–8
perception 68–9
proprioception 68
psychological effects 71
vision 69, 92
computerized tomography (CT) 66
differential diagnosis 64–6
post-operative 119
prevention 72
prognosis 71–2
treatment 70–1
Subdural haematoma, chronic 66, 84, 103
Sulphonylureas 128
Syncope 100
defaecation 102
micturition 102

Tactile sensory inattention 68
Tardive dyskinesia 34
T cell-mediated immune response 12
Temgesic (buprenorphine) 159, 160 (table)
Temporal arteritis (giant cell arteritis) 74
Terminal care 154–68
analgesic agents 159–61
pain *see* Pain
psychological aspects 166–7
symptoms 155–6
agitation 162–3
anorexia 163
anxiety 163
constipation 164
cough 161
depression 163
dyspnoea 161
excessive bronchial secretion 161
faecal impaction 164
headache 162
hypercalcaemia 165
insomnia 163
intestinal obstruction 164
monilial (Candida) infection 165

mouth problems 164–5
nausea and vomiting 163–4
odours 165–6
restlessness 162–3
ulcers 165
urinary incontinence 166
Terodiline 139
Theophylline 37
Thiamine 46
Thioridazine 55, 58, 162
Thymic cortex 12
Thyroid autoantibodies 122
Thyroid stimulating hormone 121, 123, 125
Thyrotoxicosis *see* Hyperthyroidism
Thyrotrophin-releasing hormone test 125
Thyroxine 123
T-lymphocytes 12
Tinnitus 94
Tinnitus masker 94
Todd's paralysis 66
Training/career opportunities 171–2
Tranquillizers 54–5
Transient ischaemic attacks 72–3, 95
Treatment 23–6
Tremor 77
benign essential 80
Tricyclic antidepressants 34, 57–8, 95, 101
for urinary incontinence 139
Trifluoperazine 55, 58
Trimethoprim 45

Ulcers *see also* Pressure sores
decubitus 148–53
ischaemic 148–53
malignant 165
trophic 148–53
'Unstable bladder' (detrusor instability) 138–9
Urinary catheters 144–5
Urinary continence 136–7
Urinary incontinence 80, 136–45
causes 140 (table)
drugs 142
chart 142
detrusor instability ('unstable bladder') 138–9
established 142–3
laundry service for 6
management of 144–5
investigation 143–4
neurogenic 139–40
management 145
stress incontinence 138
temporary 141–2
in terminally ill patients 166

Verapamil 29
Viscera, tumour infiltration of 156
Vision, age related changes in 86–7
Visual loss 86–92
gradual 88–90
sudden 90–2
Vitamin B complex 39 (table), 47
Vitamin B_{12} deficiency 40–1; *see also* Pernicious anaemia
bacterial overgrowth in small bowel 44
Vitamin C (ascorbic acid)
deficiency 39–40
supplements 47
Vitamin D 42, 134
deficiency *see* Osteoporosis
Voluntary organizations 5, 6, 26

Warfarin 30
Wernicke's encephalopathy 47
Wilson's disease 76